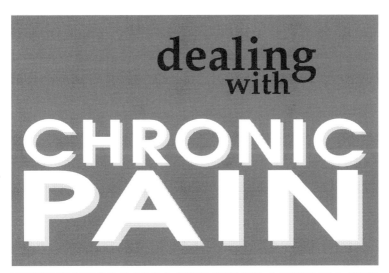

dealing with CHRONIC PAIN

THE PAIN MANAGEMENT APPROACH

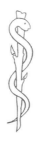

DR. JACK BARRETT
MB, BCH, BAO, FFARCSI

MARNA CAREY
MCSP

DR. GILLIAN MOORE-GROARKE
BA (HONS), PhD, NUI, REG. PSYCHOL. APsSI

ON STREAM

Published by On Stream Publications Ltd, Cloghroe, Blarney, Co. Cork, Ireland

© Dr J Barrett, M Carey, Dr G Moore-Groarke

Tel/fax: + 353 21 385798. e-mail: onstream@indigo.ie

A CIP record for this book is available from the British Library

Printed in Ireland by Sciprint, Shannon

The moral right of the authors has been asserted

ISBN 1897 685 80 7

CONTENTS

FOREWORD

Pain is the commonest symptom taking patients to see their doctor. Appropriately, the treatment of pain is taught to every doctor, as well as to every nurse and to other professionals concerned with the delivery of health care such as physiotherapy and clinical psychology. There is an increasing awareness of the widespread physical, emotional, social and economic problems that unrelieved chronic pain creates. Despite this, it simply hasn't been possible to arouse public interest and support for research into the cause and the treatment of chronic pain.

It is a fact that if pain has been unrelieved for six months or more, the chances of relieving it completely become very small indeed. However, there is still an opportunity to provide relief with effective treatment delivered with the active participation of the patient. The presence of unrelieved pain may be an enormous worry to the individual. It can lead to concerns about future health and income and to huge stresses upon family and friends. Often, understanding more about pain and why it occurs is helpful; even more helpful is knowing what can and cannot be done to help.

This book offers real help to those patients who have unrelieved pain. It will also help family members and friends understand why pain occurs, and more importantly, what can be done by the individual to help doctors and other health care workers. It is based on experience of the authors and many others throughout the world who treat pain with a combined approach: the so-called *Pain Management Programme*. This uses the skills of different pain specialists together to achieve the maximum restoration of function and return the individual with pain to as near normality as possible.

In this book you will find easy-to-read and understand explanations of how pain is transmitted within the nervous system and how the body responds to injury. There are chapters on exercise and relaxation, an explanation of some novel methods of pain relief and, most importantly, what you can do to help yourself.

The final section asks readers to look at themselves and their lifestyle and so see how simple changes in attitudes and activity can make a big difference to the levels of pain and the quality of life. There are no magic wands or miracle cures in the treatment of persistent pain, but the application of the common sense and advice found in the book will give readers a real opportunity to learn more about pain and find the way forward to a more active and fulfilling life.

J.E. Charlton
Consultant in Pain Management and Anaesthesia
Secretary, International Association for the Study of Pain
President, Pain Society (British and Irish Chapter of IASP)
Royal Victoria Infirmary
Newcastle upon Tyne
Great Britain.

INTRODUCTION

"I killed a fly today!" I cried in celebration when I realised I had the strength to cause injury to an insect which was landing on my food. To many this may seem strange, but six months ago for me it was a major milestone. My car accident took away all my strength and interest in life. For months I experienced pain so great that I believed that life was not even worth living.

My garden died with me, my relationships not enough to sustain my interest in my hobbies, my work, life itself. I lost so much weight I ended up six and a half stone; friends and family thought I could not survive, and I didn't really care whether I did or not. I had worldly goods, a wonderful husband and family who cared for me, but money could not buy me relief from pain - there was nothing to be bought that could cure me - a terrible realisation.

But the greatest lesson I have learned is that pain does not kill. I reached a stage when it was almost impossible to breathe, I was unable to talk, unable to move and the extreme pain could last for five hours before it abated to mere pain. But still I survived; the body does not give up as easily as the mind.

When painkillers in the form of drugs, coupled with other methods of pain relief such as massage and physiotherapy, were obviously not enough, a friend convinced me I should try *pain management*. The physical destruction of the body from the crash as well as the emotional aspects which I really did not acknowledge were too much for me to handle alone.

I am a typical Aquarian, nobody knows me. I am reserved and slow to ask for help; to allow people to see the real me, vulnerable or otherwise. Pain management got me to break down my barrier, that wall, that mountain which I created to protect myself from showing people I was vulnerable, not the driven businesswoman I enjoyed being. At the clinic I attended in Cork I was exposed for what I was - someone who needed help on many fronts -

there was no point in trying to fool any of them - they could see exactly what I was, and how I was hiding from them.

As each week went by my sense of humour returned, my natural aggression which I used to run my business and my home efficiently returned, and with it a sense of openness which I enjoyed seeing in myself. I started in July '96, attending each of the consultants separately before joining the group. Within six months I went from the top dose of antidepressants to 10mg a day - one tenth of the previous dose, something I thought would never be possible. In some ways I think this accident may have been good for me. I have been told I was heading for 'burn-out': working too hard, playing too hard. I would think nothing of driving to Dublin (160 miles away) for lunch and returning home the same day.

Now with the benefit of counselling, physiotherapy, group therapy and the various activities in the clinic, I can drive, the pain I feel is tolerable and I have learned to pace myself. I still cannot write, but I have been able to get back to my business, aware I must not fall into the trap of obsession with it. From the brink of destruction to the joy of living is how far I have come. I can do nothing but recommend the pages of this book and those who wrote it.

M I.B.

chapter 1

HOW WE FEEL PAIN

Pain is a common condition, not fully understood by scientists or doctors. One of the most common causes of absenteeism, it is calculated that pain, especially back pain, costs industry £400 million pounds each year in the UK. In the USA the total amounts to a staggering $100 billion when health costs and compensation are included. It is estimated that as many as thirteen percent of the population suffer from chronic pain, most commonly back and head pain, but it is also associated with a variety of diseases such as *diabetes* and *multiple sclerosis*.

Pain can be divided into **acute** pain and **chronic** pain:

Acute pain is the pain we all experience regularly, when, for example, we touch something hot or hit our finger with a hammer. It warns us that something has been injured and that we should stop whatever we are doing to prevent further injury: take away our finger from the hot plate, or to stop moving the injured part. It is therefore a protective mechanism and warns us that something is wrong, that we should react in some way to prevent further harm. We can tolerate this pain reasonably well because we know that it is warning us of danger and we expect that once the injury has healed, the pain will subside. We also expect that any treatment we have will be successful and the pain will ease with time.

By definition, **chronic pain**, on the other hand, lasts longer than three months, or beyond the normal healing time of the injury (if there was one). As the injury has healed and therefore no further warnings are needed, chronic pain would not seem to have any useful function. Very often it is resistant to pain-killers which work well for acute pain, and over time it begins to have an increasing psychological or emotional effect.

Chronic pain occurs at some stage each day and can have devastating effects on our lives, making us depressed and lacking self- confidence. We feel we are in a tunnel with very little light at the end of it. Chronic pain can affect those closest to us. Many sufferers are unable to work and their personal lives may be in ruins.

Chronic pain is best seen as a condition with a number of elements involved and manageable using an holistic approach. As it can be all-consuming it can take us over, ruining social lives. Many sufferers find it difficult to spend a whole evening at the pub or in a restaurant; others will tell you that their social lives are non-existent, leading to isolation and a feeling of being unwanted.

Pain also inhibits the use of the affected part of the body and can eventually spread to areas not originally involved. In extreme cases it can spread to most of the body. People can end up spending hours sitting in a chair or in bed 'like a zombie.'

The pain sufferer may choose to take the 'alternative' route which, if unsuccessful, leads to great despondency and further adds to the whole picture of chronic pain i.e the apparent constant failure of treatment. We often hear: "But this is the end of the 20th century, surely somebody can get rid of this pain!" Unfortunately, in many cases of chronic pain, there is no 'cure.' Patients *and* doctors can become disappointed with this lack of success of treatment and doctors can feel helpless after they have tried everything and still the patient comes back complaining of the same pain. The patient often ends up being referred to many different specialists, sometimes without success. The best advice we can often give is to stop chasing the 'cure' and learn to accept the pain and learn to live life as fully as possible. This may seem harsh to many, but much can be done for chronic pain sufferers who accept their condition and get on with their lives.

Over the past twenty years great strides have been made in research into pain. The *'gate'* theory of Drs Melzack and Wall in 1965 was the stimulus for much of this research. They proposed that pain messages passed through 'gates' on their way from the source of the pain to the brain. We now have an understanding of where these gates are and how they work.

How pain is felt

To understand how these mechanisms work it is necessary to understand how the body recognises injury and responds to it, and how the message of injury is perceived by the brain.

When a part of the body suffers damage, various chemicals are released from the site of injury. These chemicals stimulate nerves which then carry the message of injury towards the brain via 'pain nerves' to the spinal cord and up the spinal cord to the conscious brain. It is the brain that recognises pain. **If there is interruption of the message from the injured site to the brain we do not experience pain**, at least temporarily. This is a very important concept to grasp in the understanding of pain. The brain is the centre of consciousness and also of our emotions and reactions. **Pain, therefore, is a sensory** *and* **emotional experience.**

Our emotions play an important part in both the way we feel pain and also in how we react and manage pain.

Messages pass via 'small' nerves to the spinal cord where they are relayed at junctions (or gates), just like passengers on a train, to other tracks which carry them on to the brain. **Messages can be altered at these gates.** One of the ways we do it every day is by rubbing the injured area. Rubbing stimulates other 'big' nerves which travel alongside the 'small' nerves. These 'big' nerves have the effect of closing the 'gate,' thereby reducing the number of messages that pass through to the brain. **If we reduce the number of messages reaching the brain, the brain interprets this as less pain.**

The degree of injury may be the same in two cases, but the amount of pain we feel will depend on the amount of 'gate-closing' going through on the way to the brain. The more gate-closing we do, the less pain we feel. Other ways of stimulating these 'big' nerves are by acupuncture or the use of TENS (Transcutaneous Electrical Nerve Stimulator) machines. TENS machines operate electrically via pads attached to the skin. Acupuncture does it by either manual or electrical stimulation. Endorphins (the body's own, naturally produced pain-killers) also work at this site and are a very important part of our gate-closing ability.

There is nothing new in this; acupuncture has been practiced for thousands of years by the Chinese. Two thousand years ago, the Egyptians used the sting from the electric fish of the Nile as a treatment for headache. It is only recently that we have discovered how they work.

Endorphins can be generated by physical activity and also by various mental processes. Athletes are good examples of this. When marathon runners hit 'the wall' they are in extreme pain, but their training and will-power gets them through it. The release of endorphins plays a major part in this, changing the chemistry of the nerve tracks by using tricks or techniques to convince themselves they can and must go on. Pain sufferers can also learn to raise their endorphin level by physical and mental activity. This is dealt with in more detail in the chapters on physical exercise and the psychological approach of Cognitive Behavioural Therapy.

Traffic in the spinal cord is two-way. Messages pass up to the brain but they also travel down from the brain to the gates. This downward traffic acts exactly as the inward or upward traffic, i.e. it can increase the level of pain or reduce it. This can happen because the downward tracks can help to close the gates. The effect can be achieved by physical means such as exercise, but more importantly by the use of our minds: **by convincing ourselves that we can deal with the pain**. A good example of this is people who walk on hot coals without feeling the heat. It cannot be emphasised enough how important a part our minds play in our feeling of and tolerance to pain. This happens primarily at the sites of these gates.

As there is a number of ways by which we can close the gates an reduce the number of pain message to the brain, pain is often be using a combination of techniques. Drugs which act on pain may be prescribed, as well as the use of physical exercise as a therapy, and the learning of psychological techniques to help reduce the pain level.

PAIN TOLERANCE

How we react to this pain has much to do with how we can tolerate pain. We often refer to this as our **pain threshold**. This however is a misnomer, since most people's thresholds for pain are very similar. What differs is our ability to tolerate that particular pain threshold. Our pain tolerance is often conditioned by previous experience of the pain; we know it will subside over a certain time, or we know that if we take a certain drug it will ease the pain.

However, if we have had previous experience of the pain and we know that it is going to be long-lasting and maybe requires some painful treatment, we feel very different about it and our tolerance is less. It is well known that soldiers injured in battle, or sportsmen in action feel little pain initially. This is because they have the 'adrenaline' flowing and this increases their pain tolerance dramatically. The 'adrenaline' in these cases are endorphins. The soldier in battle has a high level of these endorphins and hence feels little pain. However, when time passes and he realises he will probably survive the injury, pain often develops.

CHRONIC PAIN

Research shows that when chronic pain develops, changes can take place at the spinal cord area where the gates are situated, and these changes make the nerves in the area more sensitive and reactive. This has the effect of often making the chronic pain worse than the original pain, something which many chronic pain sufferers well know. The other important factor in chronic pain is that it tends to have a significant *emotion* element. Patients with chronic pain often become depressed, not in the sense of being mentally ill, but they feel very low. Doctors therefore often prescribe anti-depressant drugs for a short period (3 months). Many of these have a pain-killing effect and thus have a dual function.

As explained in other parts of this book, chronic pain has numerous other effects on the sufferer and those who live or work with them. Carers may be unable to work due to the time necessary to look after the sufferer, and this can have a major effect on the psychological state of the patient. Such effects tend to reduce the blocking ability of the sufferer and their pain remains severe. They are unable to 'close the gate.'

Pain can also be divided into **fast pain** and **slow pain**. The fast pain is the warning which, when we prick our finger with a thorn, shoots out from the injured area and makes us react. Slow pain is the one which develops later and usually has an aching sensation. Slow pain is more complex and has more to do with our emotions and elements such as previous experience and view of outcome.

Fast pain responds well to certain pain-killers, but they may not be effective against slow pain. This will be dealt with in more detail in chapter 2. Chronic pain tends to be of the slow variety which explains why the emotional element contributes to such an extent.

An important concept is the difference between *peripheral* and *central* pain. 'Peripheral' refers to areas of the body such as the limbs and parts away from the spinal cord; 'central' refers to the brain and its extension, the spinal cord. Peripheral is the area from which the nerves come before reaching their junctions at the spine. These are the unshaded areas on the diagram.

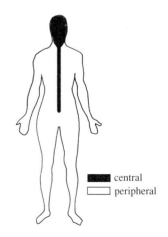

central

peripheral

Research has shown that, with certain injuries, especially those associated with chronic pain, changes can occur in the central area (the area close to the spinal cord). These changes make the affected areas (usually peripheral) more sensitive and increase the pain. They seem to set up a circle in the nervous system which can turn an acute pain, which should be short-lived, into a chronic one. Once this has occurred it is difficult to reverse. This is thought to be one of the reasons why many surgical and other peripheral treatments, such as *nerve blocks*, fail when used in isolation.

Chronic pain, therefore, must be viewed as a more complex condition than just an injury and its effects.

It is these discoveries that tell us that a comprehensive approach needs to be taken in difficult cases of unrelieved chronic pain and are the reasons why we advocate an holistic approach to the management of chronic pain.

chapter 2

MEDICAL THERAPIES

There are hundreds of different drugs, known as *analgesics*, used in the treatment of pain. They range from mild analgesics up to the strongest such as morphine. Each drug has its own characteristics and your doctor will decide which type of pain-killer is best for a particular pain.

Aspirin is still one of the most commonly used drugs for mild to moderate degrees of pain. It is also commonly used to prevent heart attacks, because it has an effect of thinning the blood, thereby helping to prevent blood-clotting. Another commonly-used drug of this type is *paracetamol*.

Both these drugs act at a site of injury and reduce the degree of inflammation that occurs, thereby reducing the number of pain messages to the brain. There are many other drugs available that act in the same way, and a pain sufferer may have to try several to find which suits best.

Pain-killers are often prescribed using the *analgesic ladder* format. Aspirin and paracetamol are on the bottom rung of the ladder, further up are drugs like codeine, and finally, at the top, are drugs such as morphine. This is one of the oldest known drugs, used for thousands of years and still used today to relieve the pain of cancer.

The drugs at the bottom of the ladder are available over the counter, while the stronger ones are available only on prescription, as they can be abused and dangerous if used without supervision of a doctor. Nevertheless, over-the-counter drugs are also dangerous if not taken as directed.

Many tablets available contain a combination of drugs such as paracetamol and codeine and sometimes *caffeine*. They may also be combined with *Non-Steroidal Anti-Inflammatory Drugs* such as *ibuprofen* or *diclofenac*, often referred to as *NSAIDS*. These are amongst the most commonly prescribed drugs for pain, especially if it is thought the pain has a muscular or joint origin. They can be very effective but are rarely suitable for long-term use because of their side-effects.

The next group of drugs up the ladder of strength are those such as *codeine*. These are commonly prescribed for moderate to severe pain. These can be very effective but they also have problems associated with their use, especially if used for a prolonged period of time. They may cause constipation and nausea. Long-term use can cause dependency and a reduction in effectiveness; this has the disadvantage of making the patient require larger doses, resulting in more side-effects and perhaps greater dependency. A vicious cycle develops.

There are drugs marketed for moderate to severe pain which avoid some of these problems. Consult your doctor for information.

Moving up the ladder to the top, *morphine* is the most commonly prescribed drug. Morphine is one of the oldest drugs known to man and is therefore well understood. It can be particularly useful for cancer pain. It is extracted from the poppy plant and was known to and used by the ancient Greeks. Morphine works at the same site as the endorphins described earlier in the book. It has the effect of raising our spirits as well as being a pain-killer. This stimulatory effect is what makes it attractive to abusers and therefore its use is strictly controlled.

Because morphine is addictive, it is not often used in chronic pain other than that associated with cancer. However, in extreme cases, it may be prescribed repeatedly if all else fails. It can be taken as a tablet or drink and is used also in injection form, often as an infusion using a drip. As it is associated with nausea and constipation, medicines need to be taken to counteract these side-effects.

The drugs described above are effective for acute pain, however they may be less effective for chronic pain as they may start to lose their effect as the body gets accustomed to them. Side-effects may prevent their long-term use, or the pain may move 'central.'

SIDE-EFFECTS

All drugs used for pain relief have side-effects and these may limit use in certain individuals. Side-effects are actions of the drug which are not its primary action, i.e. that of pain relief. However, some of these side-effects can be beneficial. The effect of thinning the blood by aspirin is a good example. This can be appropriate for certain patients but very dangerous to others. Bleeding, especially from the stomach, is a dangerous side-effect of aspirin and anybody with stomach problems such as an ulcer must avoid these drugs if at all possible.

NSAIDS work like other pain-killers by inhibiting the release of 'pain chemicals,' which are often hormones called *prostaglandins* that irritate and stimulate pain nerves at the site of injury.

These drugs, therefore, like the simple pain-killers, act at the periphery and are best for acute pain or a painful condition such as arthritis which can cause ongoing inflammation. Unfortunately, they are of less use in chronic pain because of the 'central' changes that may have occurred. The distinction between peripheral and central pain is explained in chapter 1: *'How We Feel Pain.'*

All these drugs must be taken with care because of their side-effects and the prescribed dose must not be exceeded. Stomach bleeds can be a problem with NSAIDS.

Some people might have an allergy to certain drugs, and it is important to read accompanying leaflets carefully, because many drugs are a combination of compounds and may contain one to which the taker has an allergy. If you have any doubts you must check first with your pharmacist or doctor before starting a course of treatment. You should not take over-the-counter drugs for more than a week. If symptoms do not improve, consult your doctor.

Certain drugs may even have the side-effect of causing pain. An example of this is *indomethacin*, a commonly prescribed NSAID. This can cause severe headache. Patients sometimes attend pain clinics complaining of headache and often the only treatment they need is to stop taking their 'pain-killer!'

SECONDARY ANALGESICS.

Other drugs which are not primarily pain-killers can be very useful as part of an analgesic 'cocktail.' These drugs include tranquillisers such as *Valium* to relax muscles in spasm which may be contributing to a condition such as back pain. They also can be addictive and should only be prescribed for short periods - up to six weeks. The problem with these drugs is that they take over the body's own way of doing things, in this case muscle relaxation. If you take them over a long period the body can forget how to do these things itself, and can take a long time to re-learn.

Other groups of drugs commonly used in pain clinics are anticonvulsants (usually used to treat epilepsy), and antidepressants. It may seem strange that these work for pain but they can be very effective. Anticonvulsants are used primarily for nerve pain, especially if it has a 'shooting' character. The classic example of this is *trigeminal neuralgia* or *tic douloureux*. This is a sometimes crippling pain which lasts only seconds, but is very severe and shoots across one side of the face. The face can be very sensitive, and the pain can be triggered by eating, talking or a wind blowing on the skin. The diagnosis of this condition often depends on relief using an anti-convulsant drug.

If you are put on an antidepressant drug for pain it does not necessarily mean the doctor thinks you are depressed, but because they are also useful for relieving certain pains. The most commonly used is *amitriptyline*, which is usually taken at night, as it has a side-effect of sedation and will provide the bonus of a good night's sleep. Antidepressants are used most commonly for nerve pain such as shingles, but also work on back pain, arthritis and various other conditions. They work by increasing the blocking (gate-closing) effect of the descending paths in the spinal cord.

Like all other drugs, these too have their side-effects which can be severe enough to prevent people wanting to take them. These effects can however be minimised by starting on a very low dose, and building up slowly until an effective dose is reached. This requires patience.

NON-DRUG TREATMENT

Drugs may not be the complete answer for many people, for a variety of reasons: they may not be able to tolerate the drugs or they quite reasonably do not want to be on drugs long-term. There may also not be a drug effective for their particular pain.

Many people will choose 'complementary therapies' and these are dealt with in another chapter of this book. Physical therapy and mobilisation are also very useful and are also dealt with separately in later chapters.

Medical treatments may include injections to various sites in the body or even surgery. Injections have two main purposes in pain management. First, to try to locate the source of the pain by blocking nerves to the area with local anaesthetic and seeing if this relieves the pain for a short while (This is what dentists do when they want to operate on a tooth. If the pain is relieved by the injection, other techniques can be tried to eliminate or reduce the pain). Secondly, injections can be used to block pain messages from travelling to the centre, which breaks the cycle of pain. To achieve this, a series of injections is needed, and it may require quite a number. Patience is required by all concerned.

Most commonly used injections are *epidurals, intra-articulars, sympathetic nerve blocks* (some pain can travel via 'sympathetic nerves.' These differ from the usual pain-carrying nerves, and blocking them is a well-recognised medical technique of pain control.), and more rarely, complicated injections to nerves close to the spinal cord. These require specialised techniques and equipment.

In extreme cases, surgery may be needed to get good pain relief. For example, removal of an arthritic hip and replacing it with an artificial one. Occasionally, back surgery is necessary to relieve back or leg pain caused by narrowing of the spine.

Surgery in chronic pain should usually only be contemplated as a last resort. It should not be decided on without full discussion with your doctor and the surgeon.

PAIN MANAGEMENT PROGRAMMES

Unfortunately, some patients will not get adequate relief from any treatment and the 'cure' for their pain has not yet been discovered.

Their lives are often shattered, along with their personal and work relationships. Their problems go far beyond pain, and their management is complex. One of the ways which has been shown to be effective in rehabilitation is a *pain management programme*. This is where people are taught to manage their pain and to live their lives as fully as possible. The programme uses medical, psychological and physical therapy techniques. These include exercise (to increase aerobic fitness, flexibility and strength), hydrotherapy, education (to increase body awareness), and techniques to avoid injuring the painful part further.

Psychological techniques include relaxation, pacing, goal setting and dealing with problems that may have arisen due to chronic pain.

chapter 3

THE PSYCHOLOGY OF PAIN

Perhaps the most universal form of stress encountered is pain.

Anonymous

What is the relationship between pain and the mind? What is the difference between the emotional and behavioural responses to pain? How do we measure pain and what is the relationship between stress/tension in our pain intensity ratings? What are the different ways we can think about pain? What is meant by the *Cognitive Behavioural Approach* to pain management? What does goal-setting and pacing mean in relation to pain management?

Pain is a most complex and distressing psychological experience. Chronic pain (as described in the previous chapter) can last from three months to indefinitely, despite treatment. Often there is no clear explanation why the pain is continuing. Most people with chronic pain have had an injury (or a series of injuries) and at some stage and for some reason (often psychological), the pain associated with that injury has never really gone away. The reason for this is not fully understood.

PAIN AND THE MIND

Most patients, however, tend to want to focus on their physical symptoms of pain in an attempt to find the ultimate and absolute cure. It is imperative that the psycho-social factors regarding pain are evaluated. The pain is usually felt in a part or parts of the body that are visible. Many patients with severe and prolonged symptoms of physical pain express psychological effects of the pain in terms of the physical part of the body (severe pain often leads to depression and can cause significant changes in patterns of eating, sleep and activity). The mental anguish and emotional distress that accompanies chronic pain can often produce even more suffering than the pain itself.

There are two types of psychological reaction to pain: an **emotional** reaction and a **behavioural** reaction. Such reactions are important in acute pain situations, but with chronic pain, patients feel these may be the only important features. There is considerable misunderstanding by many patients and their doctors about the psychological aspects of pain. It is as if these emotional responses and changes in behaviour somehow distort the picture portrayed by the patient who is in pain, and are different to those perceived by the doctor. This makes diagnosis difficult and can lead to inappropriate management through under-treatment or over-treatment with mood-altering drugs.

Your doctor must be fully aware of the key role of those psychological reactions to pain and provide early and effective treatment. This may take the form of anti-depressant medication if a patient is severely depressed, or referral for psychological intervention. Quick action can be of paramount importance, otherwise, treatable acute pain could progress to a chronic type and may become difficult to treat. It must also be said that when a psychologist enters the treatment scene, the patient will often react with hostility, because they feel that the medical practitioner is discussing their pain as if it were "all in the mind." This is not the case, as you will learn throughout this book, but such a reaction is not uncommon.

EMOTIONAL RESPONSES

Pain is never without an emotional response. All patients, of whatever age or circumstances, experience some distress when they are in pain. With it come feelings of fear and helplessness. The greatest fear is that your pain means that something is seriously wrong with your body, consequently patients themselves often request several M.R.I. scans to search for brain tumours, degenerative arthritis or similar conditions. Fear leads us to suspect the worst, such as seeing pain as a symptom of cancer, or thinking it could lead to paralysis or permanent disability.

As the fear becomes greater, pain usually increases. Hence many patients report feeling sick with fear. Helplessness comes from the feeling that you no longer own or can take charge of your own body, and that your pain is now dominating all your feelings and activities, preventing you from being yourself and living your own life. No matter how hard you try, the pain is always there. It is as if you are standing still at a crossroads wondering which road will provide you with a way out. Your sense of well-being becomes a thing of the past: there is little to look forward to and little comfort.

These emotional reactions usually increase the sensitivity of injured tissues, and pain increases. Pain then feeds on anxiety which in turn feeds on pain. The more distressed you become the more you will become depressed. Depression adds to mental anguish, and both pain-relieving and anxiety-relieving medication will often be administered.

Chronic pain goes hand-in-hand with complex emotional responses. Depression, negative or morbid thought patterns, even suicidal thoughts, lead to a semi-vegetative or sedentary lifestyle in many patients. Activity decreases to minimal levels and patients soon lose interest in themselves and their surroundings. Weight gain can result which fuels depression and inactivity. The disease then becomes chronic pain. Because of such symptoms, advice from a dietician is often required for appropriate patient care.

BEHAVIOURAL RESPONSES

The behavioural responses to pain are movements, postures and body expressions we use when we are re-experiencing pain. These are features that a doctor and physiotherapist observe and use to assess the severity of pain. They can be used to arrive at a diagnosis and as a guide to planned therapy intervention. Such interventions will be discussed in later chapters.

Facial expression, or other pain body language such as a guarded or hunched posture, sitting or standing with a noticeable stiffness, or holding or grabbing the pain area are also behavioural responses to pain. Such responses are a way of communicating to others how much pain is felt. Research has shown that medical personnel usually respond to such signs by administering pain-relieving medication. However, relying on these behavioural expressions alone is not enough. Ironically, the so-called 'difficult' patient who verbally moans and groans the most about his/her pain will be most likely to receive prompt attention and to be given relief.

MEASURING PAIN

Although pain is basically a subjective experience it can be measured, but with some difficulty and within limits. The first stage of a pain management programme shows patients how to record their pain and to find out how and why it varies at different times. The first task is to spend a week recording the amount of pain felt over the day. This does not mean dwelling on the pain, but rather estimating how much it hurts at different times. Patients rate their pain on a 5 point scale. 0 when no pain is experienced, and 5 is classified as excruciating pain or the worst possible pain you can imagine.

Example of Week 1 Pain Rating Diary (using a 5 point scale)

MONDAY						
TIMES	**SCORE**	**1**	**2**	**3**	**4**	**5**
08.00	2					
10.00	2					
12.00	3					
02.00	3					
04.00	4					
06.00	4					
08.00	5					
10.00	3					

TUESDAY

TIMES	SCORE	1	2	3	4	5
08.00	2					
10.00	3					
12.00	3					
02.00	3					
04.00	4					
06.00	4					
08.00	4					
10.00	3					

WEDNESDAY

TIMES	SCORE	1	2	3	4	5
08.00	3					
10.00	2					
12.00	4					
02.00	3					
04.00	4					
06.00	4					
08.00	5					
10.00	2					

THURSDAY

TIMES	SCORE	1	2	3	4	5
08.00	2					
10.00	2					
12.00	2					
02.00	3					
04.00	2					
06.00	4					
08.00	2					
10.00	3					

FRIDAY						
TIMES	**SCORE**	**1**	**2**	**3**	**4**	**5**
08.00	2					
10.00	2					
12.00	3					
02.00	3					
04.00	4					
06.00	4					
08.00	3					
10.00	3					

SATURDAY						
TIMES	**SCORE**	**1**	**2**	**3**	**4**	**5**
08.00	3					
10.00	3					
12.00	3					
02.00	4					
04.00	4					
06.00	2					
08.00	2					
10.00	2					

SUNDAY						
TIMES	**SCORE**	**1**	**2**	**3**	**4**	**5**
08.00	2					
10.00	2					
12.00	3					
02.00	3					
04.00	2					
06.00	2					
08.00	3					
10.00	2					

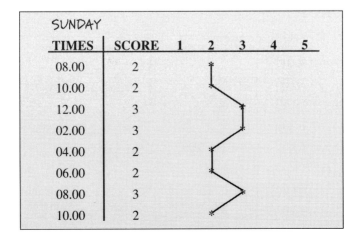

WHAT RECORDING CAN TELL YOU

Most patients insist that there is no variation in their pain, it just hurts all the time. But when they record it in this sort of detail over the day they are surprised to find that the pain intensity is generally higher as the day goes on. For many people pain increases throughout the day, with a high point at about 8pm, as can be seen in some of the graphs.

It is also important to record tension ratings and their consequent effects on pain. Tension is best defined as a feeling of emotional strain and a general disturbance in one's sense of well-being. Generally, the higher the tension ratings the greater the pain intensity. Tension is also rated on a 5 point scale where 0 is no tension and 5 is unbearable tension.

Contributing factors are assessed by asking patients what they are doing at the time of recording the pain and tension. They are also asked to record what they are thinking, to assess any negative thought patterns which may in fact be contributing to increased pain/tension ratings. There is generally a strong correlation between high pain intensity ratings and high tension recordings. Again, as in pain intensity ratings, tension levels usually increase and peak throughout the latter part of the day.

The following example is from a patient whose young family is very dependent on her. It is obvious that when the children return from school, her tension increases. This is quite common in patients suffering from chronic pain. The desire to opt out of family life is all too tempting as you can see from what this patient is thinking when recording her pain and tension.

SAMPLE PAIN AND TENSION RECORD

Time	(0-5) Pain Rating	(0-5) Tension Rating	What am I doing?	What am I thinking?
9am	2.3	2	Having breakfast	Busy day ahead: housework, shopping etc.
1pm	2.4	2.5	Preparing dinner	Finding that it is taking so long.
5pm	4	3	Dinner, housework, children have returned from school.	Finding the invasion of the family difficult to cope with, everyone making demands.
8pm	4	3.2	Watching TV	Feeling I would love to be alone.
10pm	4.3	4.2	Preparing lunches and setting breakfast table.	Fear of being unable to sleep once again tonight.

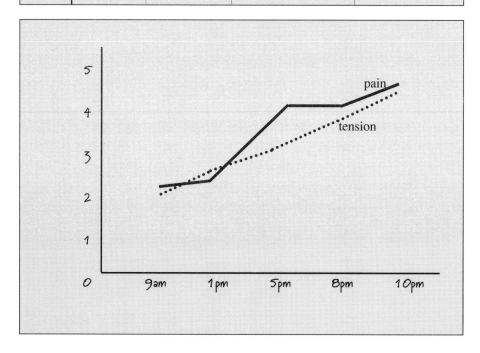

WAYS OF THINKING ABOUT PAIN

Most people with chronic pain feel that it is unfair, and experience depression, irritability, despair, frustration, anger and isolation. It is important to understand that it is not just pain that influences how you feel. The way you see yourself, the past and the future, all play a big part in making you feel the way you do. Negative thinking prevents us from trying increased activity levels. Negative thinking patterns can easily become habitual. Furthermore, like ways of behaving, some ways of thinking can become unhelpful and like all habits, unhelpful thinking patterns take an effort to change.

At first, you may find it hard to see how to change the ways you think and feel. Many people believe that they have no control over their thoughts and feelings and that they are just made like that. Yet, in the past, you probably changed your mind about something, or kept your temper when you felt angry. Most probably you changed your mind about something after listening to yourself and talking things through with yourself. Worry, anxiety and panic reinforces the pain response, so therefore it is important to address ways of coping with negative thought patterns as part of any pain management programme.

At times of difficulty ask yourself: "Am I being realistic about the risk?" For instance, if your pain is increasing, do you find yourself worrying that it is some undiagnosed and serious disease, and start picturing yourself bed-ridden, helpless or worse? Alternatively, do you think of all the other possibly less serious reasons for it worsening, and what you *are* able to do?

Focusing on the things you fear such as collapsing, breaking down in public or losing control all increase pain intensity ratings. It is not uncommon for patients with chronic pain to experience severe panic attacks. Your confidence is also important when it comes to dealing with fears and worries about pain. Confidence comes from doing something well, recognising it, remembering it and telling yourself and (other people) about it. Coping with your pain, and carrying on as normal a life as possible despite it, are things you know how to do well. It is more important to cope with the pain by recognising your limits than by fighting it. Stopping to think and plan, instead of panicking, is a success in itself. If you expect yourself to manage perfectly, you will often be disappointed.

It is a good idea to think of some situation around your pain and identify your feelings regarding that situation. Secondly, identify your negative thoughts and what could you do to change them.

Example taken from a patient suffering from chronic pain for 15 years before joining a pain management programme:

Situation	Feelings	Negative thoughts
Doctor said "You will be in a wheelchair by the time you're 50."	*Despair, anger, resignation.*	*What is the point in trying? Why me? It is so unfair!*

From the above example it is clear that this young man had two choices. He could have become resigned to the statement that he would end up in a wheelchair, which would have been a negative response. Or, a more positive response would have been to play a more active role in his own recovery by learning to manage his pain within his own limits.

Once the feelings of anger, despair and resignation are spoken about and dealt with, new coping strategies such as vigilance (i.e. facing up to the pain) rather than avoidance (hoping the problem would disappear, and an even more obsessive desire to find the cure) could be taken on board.

PAIN MANAGEMENT–THE COGNITIVE BEHAVIOURAL APPROACH

The *Cognitive Behavioural Therapy* (CBT) approach to pain management is very much a multi-dimensional approach, moving away from the standard medical treatment. Patients who enter pain management programmes stress their desires to no longer be treated as a set of walking symptoms. The CBT model looks at not just the physical symptoms but also the emotional, behavioural and cognitive (perceptual) dimensions of a patient's pain.

CBT is based on five basic assumptions and requires the intervention of a psychologist.

1 Patients' responses to pain are based on their past or learned experiences of pain. Often, during a psychological interview, patients reveal a history of chronic pain within their families. When asked if they can identify any advantages to their lives living with chronic pain, they invariably list increased social support (attention-seeking) as the most common advantage to their pain.

2 Stress increases pain and subsequent physiological responses. Stress management and coping skills play an important part in a pain management programme, as psychological responses to pain increase the number of requests for anxiolytic (anxiety-reducing) medication.

3 As the pain intensity increases due to psychosomatic (stress-related) symptoms, a greater need for medical intervention is required. Often, no true organic cause can be found at the time the patient applies for treatment. One patient complained of a persistent pain in her chest which turned out to be a panic attack. Similar panic attacks were a manifestation of living in a difficult domestic situation, and, in particular, her relationship with her husband.

4 Treatment assesses a patient's environmental factors, their emotions (thoughts and feelings), behaviours, stress levels and physiological responses. The psychological impact/symptoms of chronic pain include depression, anxiety, panic, weight loss/gain, disturbed sleep patterns, loss of libido, stressful interpersonal relationships, reduced self-esteem, and poor quality of life.

5 Patients are taught to take an active role in their own recovery. By taking this on board, the patient is learning, with the help of a psychologist, how to monitor the internal or external events that are associated with increased pain ratings, and to prevent or reduce symptoms of pain by employing relaxation and other coping skills.

The goals of the psychologist are:

* to help patients become problem solvers.

* to monitor patients' thought progression in such a way that they can overcome helplessness and associated negative thinking, and learn new coping skills to adapt to their new limits.

Treatment is based on education, not just of the patient, but also their partners and family. Pain management programmes invite all family members to attend, to share how they feel about living with somebody in chronic pain. The session also acts as a forum for the family to open up about their anger and resentment regarding the changes in their lifestyle, and the greater burden often placed upon them.

Relaxation Skills training plays a vital role in the CBT model and this will be discussed in detail in a later chapter. Patients are taught to plan for future events and to prepare for setbacks. All the skills taught through CBT have been shown to reduce pain behaviour, disease activity, pain intensity ratings, the need for social support, psychological disability, the need for psychiatric intervention (including anti-depressant medication), and the rate of relapse. Two important elements of the CBT model also include goal-setting and pacing.

GOAL-SETTING AND PACING

As each person with chronic pain will face different problems, it is important that you should first identify the problems you want to deal with and the goals you want to achieve. Whatever your goals may be, you are going to have to make some changes in the way you have been living. It is best to start with easy goals to gradually build up confidence.

The fear of pain and of doing more damage will hold you back. Do not be afraid to look for reassurance from medical personnel you are working with. Do a little to begin with. Goals will take time to achieve - you must be patient with yourself.

☀ List your reasons for trying.

☀ Record your progress.

☀ Reward yourself.

☀ Do not be afraid to ask for help.

Pacing means slowing down in all your activities, not just activities that are difficult, and learning to recognise your new physical and mental limitations. While the physiotherapist works through physical goals with the patient, the psychologist focuses on goals of well-being. A useful exercise is to set out a hierarchy of goals as a form of commitment to yourself. The following example indicates not only what these goals might be, but also a realistic time frame.

HIERARCHY OF PSYCHOLOGICAL GOAL-SETTING AND PACING

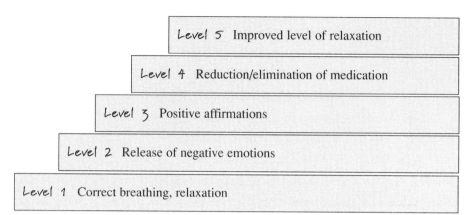

Level 5 Improved level of relaxation

Level 4 Reduction/elimination of medication

Level 3 Positive affirmations

Level 2 Release of negative emotions

Level 1 Correct breathing, relaxation

Increasing in intensity, each level represents one month

The role of the psychologist, and indeed the role of all health professionals on a pain management programme, becomes that of a consultant. Rather than being expected to cure the patient, the health professional's task and especially the task of the psychologist, is to foster the development of self-reliance in the patient. The psychological intervention serves to facilitate a very important transition for the patient from **being treated** to **treating oneself**. As mentioned already, this attitude creates less dependency of the patient on the medical team. When the patient is faced with a similar problem in the future, he or she recognises the psychological dimension to pain and the effect a change in attitude/behaviour may have in helping to alleviate or solve the problem. The psychology of pain is most definitely based on the "mens sano corporo sano" philosophy where it is said that "a healthy mind is in a healthy body." If unsuccessful, a patient can always return to any of the pain management team for assistance or relearning of skills. The emphasis is on managing the pain, rather than searching for a so-called 'cure.'

chapter 4

THE IMPORTANCE OF EXERCISING AND PACING TECHNIQUES IN MANAGING PAIN

The importance of exercising and pacing techniques in the management of pain cannot be over-emphasised. Immobility may cause pain to increase. It is necessary to move the affected muscles and joints to prevent any further decline in strength, flexibility and aerobic fitness. A regular gentle exercise programme can help increase your mobility and fitness, allowing more activities and tasks to be achieved within the day.

People with a chronic condition are often frightened to move a painful area as it may cause a 'flare-up.' This is not the case. Initially an immobile joint or tight muscle will object to moving again, but, within limitations and if practiced regularly, a degree of the original mobility can be regained. This applies especially to those affected areas of the body which have become stiff purely due to lack of use - not due to injury.

If confined to bed, the muscle groups in the body will suffer some wasting. This means they lose power to move the joints and support the body against gravity. A sportsman who has suffered injury to a thigh muscle will lose strength within 24 hours due to inhibition of that muscle. Inhibition is a prevention of muscle contraction due to pain messages being sent from the brain which tell the muscle to avoid the pain which would result from movement.

In the case of a non-sports injury, wasting will also occur, and total bed-rest not only causes decreased power of the injured muscle groups, but weakness of all other areas too.

The pain will be reduced by bed-rest if the muscle is allowed to weaken and therefore relax, but by the time you are able to move again the damage has already been done. It is therefore important to start moving early; even if you are confined to bed for 24 hours you can move the unaffected areas. In the initial stages of bed-rest, it has been found that mobilising an equal amount of time to resting shows maximum improvement in movement and reduction of pain.

For the body to function effectively it must have mobile joints and strong, flexible muscles which are supplied by an efficient blood and nerve supply and connected by a network of ligaments.

In the chronic pain patient, an enormous decrease in muscle flexibility is found due to shortening of the affected muscle in response to pain or from protecting a painful area and holding it in a contracted position.

Once the spasm has been controlled, it is necessary to regain or improve the muscle's stretching capacity. This is done by a number of stretching exercises which will be taught to you by a physiotherapist and must be done daily and on an ongoing basis to achieve improvement. It is important to stretch both upper and lower limb muscle groups, even if you have no pain in those areas, because they will have been affected due to the alteration of your body's mechanics in response to pain. Illustrated at the end of the book are the common muscle stretches and some gentle back and neck exercises which can be done under the supervision of an approved practitioner. These stretches will be more effective if done when you are warm; after a warm shower or bath is a good time. Never stretch a muscle when cold, as you may end up with further injury.

To improve muscular strength you do not need to attend a gym and 'pump iron.' There are two ways you can improve muscle strength:

- ☀ By **dynamic resisted movement** - when the muscle is contracting and moving against a resistance.
- ☀ By **static resisted movement** - when a muscle is contracting in one position against a resistance.

Both types of strength are necessary to gain good function from a muscle.

Dynamic movement is the main strength necessary in everyday activities - lifting a baby, vacuuming and sweeping or digging - whereas **static muscle power** is used in such activities as drying your hair, holding a pen or reading a book. Both dynamic and static muscle contractions have to work in conjunction with each other: when lifting objects such as a box or a baby, the muscles of the back have to fix your spine in an appropriate position to enable your arms and legs to lift effectively.

In order to strengthen a muscle you must work against a resistance, which can be anything from gravity to a gym weight. Increasing the resistance you work against, or the amount of repetitions you carry out, can increase the strength. Often with chronic pain, people find a lighter resistance with more repetitions easier than lifting a heavy weight a lesser number of times.

If you suffer from nerve compression or a traction injury, you may find that repetitive type movements in the affected area cause flare-ups. Therefore, it is not advisable to carry out too many repetitions - it is very important to pace yourself when starting an exercise programme. We will discuss this later in the chapter.

There are many commercial weights and resistance accessories available on the market but you need not spend time or money unnecessarily. A small bag with weighed sand, salt or sugar will do the trick. It is very important that if you are going to commence a weight programme that it is done under supervision of an appropriate practitioner. When you first start an exercise programme you will probably need no weights. The counter resistance from gravity will be sufficient, especially if you have had a period of inactivity or are unfit. Illustrated in chapter 8 are some general strengthening exercises, which must be supervised and progressed by your practitioner.

To increase mobility of a joint it must move through a range of movement. Each joint in the body has an accepted range of movement, but it is unusual in an adult to have full movement, due to ongoing wear and tear, postural deviations, shortening of muscle groups and the constant stress of having to stand upright. It is therefore important to remember that when you start on a mobility programme, you will not be able to move your shoulder through the same range as that of a professional tennis player, or that your spine will flex like a gymnast. Your goals must be realistic for your age and fitness.

Mobility exercises require no resistance, the aim being to move the joint through as great a range as possible without causing undue discomfort. These exercises should be carried out after a stretching regime and before a strengthening or weight programme. You will often find that your mobility is restricted because another joint or group of joints are not functioning properly. For example, your shoulder movement may be limited if you have suffered a neck injury due to immobility of your shoulder blades, neck and upper back areas. Often, you will find that mobilising one area will cause discomfort in another region, so you must not push too hard. Try to mobilise the stiffest area first, that is the neck and upper back, and then the shoulder blades, as in the above example.

Most exercises will not just mobilise a joint or strengthen a muscle, they work in conjunction to perform a task; you may find you have to improve your muscle strength before you can move a specific joint. For example, if your deltoid muscle on your shoulder is weak, you will not be able to move the shoulder through its available range. This also applies to the muscles of the spine and neck.

COMBINED EXERCISE AND AEROBIC ACTIVITIES

The perfect complement to strengthening and flexibility exercises is a combined exercise and aerobic programme, which is necessary to improve co-ordination, endurance and circulation.

Aerobic exercise is any exercise for which the body uses oxygen. These exercises will condition your heart and lungs, thus improving circulation and endurance. They usually require a number of muscle groups and areas to work together, therefore improving co-ordination. Examples of aerobic exercise are swimming, cycling, treadmills and walking. It is important that the aerobic exercise you choose is compatible with your age, lifestyle and fitness.

To improve aerobic fitness it is necessary to include one or a combination of the above activities in your schedule for 20 - 30 minutes, 3 - 5 times a week.

Pulse-taking is an effective way to find out whether your aerobic exercise programme is working effectively and that your fitness is improving. The goal of aerobic fitness is to reach your *target heart rate* (THR) for at least 20 minutes. The chart below shows the average THR for your age (don't be disappointed if your heart rate is higher, this will be due to any period of reduced activity or bed-rest you may have had). Immediately after exercise, take your pulse on the wrist, count for 15 seconds and multiply by four. This will give you your heartbeats per minute. *Always take your pulse after the same length of exercise, for example 20 minutes.*

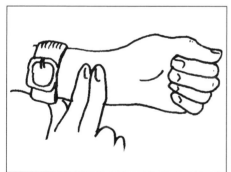 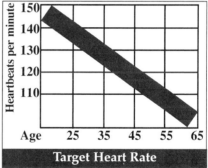

You will notice as you progress with your exercise programme that your heartbeat will decrease. This is a sign of improved overall fitness. You will start to feel generally better, with more energy and better motivation. This is partly due to the release of endorphins, which is similar to the effect runners feel after exercise and which makes them want to do it regularly.

When choosing an aerobic activity, it is very important that you pace yourself and set realistic targets. You must progress your exercise programme slowly and commence with one activity, only introducing a new one when you are managing your initial activity with undue stress or fatigue.

Here is a suggested programme

WEEK 1   Walking 10 minutes, 3 times a week.
Note distance and pulse.

WEEK 2   Walking 10 minutes, 3 times a week.
Aim: To increase distance covered.

WEEK 3   Walking 15 minutes, 3 times a week.
Aim: To increase distance every second day.

WEEK 4   Walking 15 minutes, twice a week; add one new activity,
e.g. Aqua-aerobics, Treadmill, Cycling for 10 minutes
a.week. Progress as for walking.

If any activity causes a flare-up, reduce or stop and concentrate on other methods of exercise.

WARM-UPS

Stretching your muscles and softening your discs prevent further injury. The most effective warm-ups are stretching exercises and some gentle mobilising exercises for your spine and neck - this will already be part of your programme. You must ensure that you do them immediately before and after aerobic exercise. Do not get cold after stretching, as that defeats the whole purpose of the warm-up. It is important that you wear appropriate clothing, to keep the muscles warm, and that you start exercising immediately after the warm-up.

HYDROTHERAPY

Swimming can sometimes cause discomfort due to excessive pressure on the neck and lower back. It is better to perform exercises in water and use a float for gentle leg strengthening, rather than trying to complete lengths of free-style and breaststroke. Using a snorkel minimises any stress on the neck, and allows strengthening of both the upper and lower limbs.

Many of the exercises performed on dry land can be done in the water; this gives the added advantage of the weightless environment together with the resistance of the water when displacing it with an arm or a leg. To increase resistance in water you can use floats or specially made dumbells. There are special neck floats available which allow your neck to be supported whilst exercising your lower limbs. Walking in the water in itself is very good aerobic exercise. This can be varied by moving sideways, backwards etc. which combines fitness and co-ordination.

Hydrotherapy must be supervised by a qualified practitioner.

CYCLING

It is more beneficial to start a cycling programme on a static exercise bike than a conventional pushbike. This is because the environment on the open road is not controlled, and contains bumps, potholes, stray dogs etc. It is therefore advisable to start cycling at home or in the gym and, as you increase your fitness and co-ordination, take to the open road, avoiding hills if possible, as they will cause excess strain, particularly in the upper limb muscle groups. Try to keep your pace even throughout the exercise programme.

TREADMILL

Using a treadmill in a supervised environment is important when beginning an aerobic programme. When suffering from chronic pain the fear of being jostled and walking on uneven ground is normal, so it may be beneficial to start your exercise programme on a treadmill in the gym and progress to walking outside. It is better to increase your distance then to increase the resistance. If you increase your distance within a fixed time you are certainly improving your aerobic fitness. It is important to wear the correct clothing as discussed below in the *Walking* section.

WALKING

For many people this is the most available option as it is on your doorstep, free and acceptable. It is particularly important when starting a walking programme to have the correct equipment:

- A pair of well-cushioned shoes which will act as shock-absorbers and reduce the stress through your spine and the rest of your body.
- Comfortable, loose clothing which will allow you freedom of movement and protect you from the sun and rain.
- A wristwatch or stopwatch to assess your progress.

Increasing your distance in the same amount of time shows you are improving aerobically. For example, walking 5km in 40 minutes is an improvement in walking 4km in 40 minutes. You may find it helpful to chart your progress on paper.

It is very important that before you embark on any form of aerobic exercise that you warm up your body.

PACING AND GOAL-SETTING

Taking an active role in managing your chronic pain is not just a case of starting an exercise programme. It is of the utmost importance that you learn to pace yourself, set realistic goals and plan to avoid flare-ups.

You have heard the term *pacing and goal-setting* in previous chapters. It is impossible to over-stress how important they are to your overall management. Pacing is important in every aspect of your daily life whether washing the dishes or carrying out an exercise programme.

We all know that when our pain level is lower, we push ourselves too hard to catch up and get things done. We want to prove to our family and friends that we can still manage to do things as we did prior to the chronic pain. The result of pushing too hard is an increase in symptoms, or a flare-up which returns you to square one. You may end up needing to increase medication and becoming generally frustrated believing you are not going to achieve your goals. This is why pacing is essential for progress.

* Consider an activity which after some time causes an increase in symptoms - walking, sitting, housework.
* Time how long it takes for the activity to cause your pain to increase. Do this on 3 consecutive days.
* Total the number of minutes or seconds, and divide by 3 which will give you a daily average. Take this total and halve it.

This is the amount of time you should participate in this activity. Do not be tempted to do it for longer because you have no pain. This is the whole concept of pacing - to cease an activity *before* flare-up. This formula can be used in any situation from the treadmill in the gym to reading a book. For the formula to work effectively you must progress your time gradually.

PACING AND GOAL-SETTING FORMULA

WALKING	TIME
Day 1	10 min
Day 2	12 min
Day 3	14 min
Total	**36 min**
Daily Average	**12 min**
Half	**6 min**
	This is your target ti

days, re-assess the time it takes for you to become uncomfortable an activity and note whether the time has increased from the initial assessment. If it has, use the formula to calculate how much increase in time is necessary. This may seem complicated but once you start to use it and chart your progress it will become second nature.

You do not always have to use the formula to control your activities. It would not be feasible to time every activity by the minute during your day. Using common sense you can prevent flare-ups by planning the day, knowing your limitations and modifying your environment. Many activities we carry out daily are unnecessary or can be done in a different way. Old habits die hard. Do your really need to dust the living room daily? Stand back and take a look at your day - you may be able to make a few simple alterations to your routine which will make life easier.

AT HOME

- If you have stairs, plan how often you need to go up and down; minimise the amount of trips.
- Start using rice and pasta as an alternative to potatoes.
- Use a duvet instead of sheets and blankets.
- Use your pacing techniques for activities such as ironing, mowing the lawn, sweeping the floor. It doesn't matter if only half of it is done. If you pace yourself, you will be able to complete the task later, or the following day, instead of pushing yourself into so much discomfort that for the next two days you are unable to do anything.

Planning your environment is very important. A few alterations to your home could reduce pain levels.

- Ensure that objects you use daily are accessible - dishes should not be in overhead or low-level cupboards. They should be stored at waist level to reduce the amount of muscle work and joint stress.

☀ Work surfaces, whether in the kitchen or garden shed, must be at the correct height for you. If they are too high, use a footstool or telephone book to raise your height. This applies to sinks and ironing boards as well. If there is a table which is more appropriate, cover it with newspaper or plastic and use it as your work surface.

☀ If you are more comfortable sitting than standing, use a bean-bag table, and carry out tasks such as food preparation on your lap.

☀ Have a small stepladder available to reach into higher cupboards.

☀ Balance the weight you are carrying - equal weight of shopping bags in each hand.

If you have difficulty bending or reaching, there are many aids to help pick objects up from the floor or from a high cupboard - some for putting on stockings and socks too. If you suffer from weakness or pain in the hands, there are aids to help you open jars, turn knobs etc. Use long-handled tools e.g. paint rollers, feather dusters, garden shears.

If driving, ensure that your seat is at the correct height. You can raise your position by placing a piece of foam rubber on top. Most new cars have lumbar supports, but if yours does not, ensure that you have a lumbar roll or cushion in the small of the back. Do not drive sitting back too far from the wheel as stretching for the pedals increases muscular strain.

If you are working at a desk, make sure that you have a firm supportive chair. If it does not have lumbar support, use a lumbar roll or a small, rolled-up towel. Ensure that the chair is at the correct height, i.e. feet flat on the ground and knees at hip level or slightly higher - you can alter this by using a footstool. Your eyes should be level with the computer screen, and the keyboard just below the level of the elbows so that your wrists are sloping down slightly.

ERGONOMICS (BODY MECHANICS)

You will frequently hear this word by your physiotherapist. It is a very important part of a self-management programme because, by following the guidelines, you will reduce stress to the body and prevent further injury.

Ergonomics, when used in conjunction with good body mechanics, help to give our bodies support and prevent continual repetitive strain.

Body mechanics simply means using the body as a machine as effectively as possible. Your body will function at its best if it is well greased and oiled, flexible, fit and strong. This is why an exercise programme is paramount to allowing your body to perform well.

LYING AND SLEEPING

- ☀ **Do not** sleep or lie on a soft bed or sofa. Your spine and neck will be unsupported and this may result in back and neck strain.
- ☀ **Do** sleep on a firm mattress with an orthopedic pillow (or a small towel rolled up and placed between your pillow and pillow case to support the curve in your neck). You may sleep on your side with your knees bent up if you suffer discomfort in your lower back. In this position, try putting a small pillow between your knees and a small rolled-up towel under your waist. This will help to keep your spine in good alignment. You may sleep on your back with pillows under your knees and a towel under your lower back. This will help to reduce stress on your spine.
- ☀ **Do** always get out of bed by rolling on your side, bending your knees up towards your chest. As your legs come over the side of the bed push yourself into the sitting position using your elbow and hand. To lie down, do the opposite. You must form a habit of this, as it prevents any excessive rotation of the spine.

STANDING

✷ **Do not** slouch or spend long periods of time bent forward from the waist with the legs straight.

✷ **Do not** wear high heels.

✷ **Do** bend your knees to prevent slouching. For example, when you are cleaning your teeth or in the shower, position your head squarely over your body.

✷ **Do** change positions frequently and alter the position of your back by standing with one foot up on a box or telephone book and changing after a few minutes. Sit or lie for short periods of time if possible.

WALKING

✷ **Do not** walk in high heels.

✷ **Do not** carry heavy weights.

✷ **Do not** carry heavy shoulder bags.

✷ **Do not** walk with the head, shoulders and lower back bent forwards.

✷ **Do** wear good supportive flat shoes.

✷ **Do** balance weights by carrying two similar ones on either side, or use a small rucksack.

✷ **Do** try to maintain the 3 natural curves in your back by keeping your chin tucked in and reducing the curve in your lower back. (*see p. 59*)

SITTING

✷ **Do not** slump.

✷ **Do not** sit in a chair that is too soft or too far from your work.

✷ **Do not** do exercise that involves arching your lower back.

✷ **Do** sit with a lumbar roll or small towel to support your lower back.

✷ **Do** sit in a chair low enough to place both feet flat on the floor or knees slightly higher than the hips. This can be done using a stool or telephone book if you cannot alter the height of the chair.

✷ **Do** raise your reading materials to eye level using a box or books.

✷ **Do** alter your position - this is helpful in reducing stress on the body.

LIFTING

Correct lifting is important even if you have not suffered a back or neck injury, because the load through the spine determines how many other muscle groups and joints have to come into play to allow the spine to function. It makes sense that using the back efficiently will lessen the work of other areas whilst lifting. The lower back acts as a pivot. If lifting is carried out correctly, the weight of the spine in supporting is minimal. If used incorrectly, the pivot has to support both the weight of the body and the load.

These principles apply whether the load is 20kg or 2kg. Lifting a light weight repeatedly can also cause problems.

Before we discuss the principles of good lifting, let us put some thought into problem-solving. Think about the load you are going to lift:

How much does it weigh?
How large a surface area has it?
Where are you taking it?
Is the pathway clear?

Test the weight first by lifting it a small distance towards you. You will know if it is too heavy. If the weight is too heavy or too large, get help. Remember, this could be the straw that breaks the camel's back. It may take more time to get help but could prevent injury.

If there is no-one to help, look for a mechanical alternative: a trolley, hoist or wheelbarrow. Always push, do not pull. Ensure the pathway through which you are carrying your load and your destination is clear.

PREVENTING HIGH AND LOW PROBLEMS

Lifting from above the shoulder level can be very dangerous, as the strain through your lumbar spine is much greater than lifting from the waist level.

Try to get as close to the weight as possible by using a stepladder or footstool, and pull the weight towards you to test it. Mentally plan the lift, ie, *down the steps, turn and walk across the floor.* Ensure your destination is clear.

Try to organise your environment so that most of your lifting is at waist height. The less overhead and low lifting you do, the less chance you have of increasing your pain. If you are at work, talk to colleagues or the occupational health and safety officer to help solve any problems.

GOOD LIFTING PRINCIPLES

- Get close to the load. Stand with your feet apart at shoulder width with toes turned slightly out.
- Bend your knees, *never bend from the waist*, and grip the load firmly.
- Maintain the 3 natural curves in your back.
- Tighten your abdominal muscles.
- Lift by using your strong leg muscles to straighten the knees, avoid any twisting.
- Keep the load close to your body.
- Set down the load by keeping your back straight and bending your knees slowly.

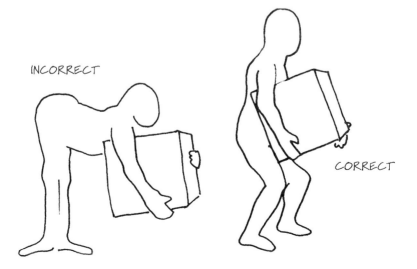

INCORRECT

CORRECT

If you enlist help to lift an object, try to find somebody near your own height and build. To avoid misunderstandings, decide on who gives clear instructions, as uncoordinated lifting could cause more problems than lifting on your own. Instructions should be straightforward: *"on the count of three we will lift 1, 2, 3."* Make sure you both know your pathway and destination.

POSTURE

Posture is always affected to some degree by chronic pain. It is controlled from a mechanism based in a part of the brain called the *cerebellum* and, in the normal run of things, if the body tilts too far backwards or forwards, this will automatically be corrected by different groups of muscles contracting.

If the back or the neck has been injured or is suffering from some long-term stress, some of these muscles will have gone into spasm and therefore their contraction may have altered the shape of the spine. If one particular area of the spine is altered, for example the lower back area, there is a knock-on effect into the middle back and neck. There will therefore be further compensation needed to keep the body in the functional upright position. You may even find that the position of the pelvis is altered. This is the reason that so many people complain of pain secondary to their initial problem.

Certain groups of muscles will have to work in a way that they were not designed to. They can therefore become very tired resulting in a sensation of burning pain. This can happen in different parts of the spine, e.g. the left lower back and right neck area due to the alteration of the spinal curves. People often complain of headaches due to compression at the top of the spine.

Pain can occur in the hips, knees and feet due to an alteration in weight-bearing. This is because the centre of gravity has been thrown off-line and, therefore, more strain is being taken through particular areas. If you imagine a plumb-line from the head down through the base of the skull, the lower back, the pelvis and falling between the feet, the body is balanced and does not have to work too hard to stay upright against gravity. If, after injury, the posture is altered, the centre of gravity can be thrown off line either sideways, forwards or backwards. This means there will be excessive strain through groups of muscles and certain joints. It is therefore very important to build up an awareness of your posture and do as much as possible to correct it. If your posture improves you will most likely suffer less discomfort.

The most effective way to assess posture is by looking in a mirror; by standing sideways you will get the best aspect. Normal posture is an 'S' shape. You will find that posture deteriorates with age, so your posture may not have been perfect even when you were pain-free. Most people with chronic pain have a tendency to have a poking chin, a rounded middle back and shoulders, and a flattened lower back. Although in some cases you find an exaggerated lower back curve and flattened middle back and neck areas, this is often predisposed by the original posture and, of course, by the type of injury. Someone with chronic pain tends not to move the painful areas, therefore these patterns become fixed and some areas particularly stiff.

The Three Natural Curves of the Back	Posture

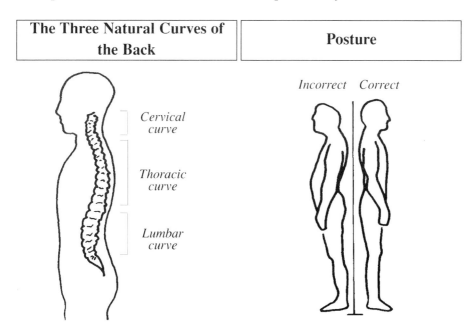

Cervical curve

Thoracic curve

Lumbar curve

Incorrect   Correct

body to function well, posture must be aligned. If you have pain in the or shoulders, your posture will most certainly be affected. To change your postural pattern you must move the stiff joints, improve the flexibility of the muscles and increase the power of the muscle groups especially the areas which have to support the body against gravity. Your exercise programme will encompass these.

There is one other very important factor to consider when talking about posture, and that is the position of the pelvis. The pelvis acts as a pivot and a base from which the spine rises. **For the spine to be in the correct position the pelvis must be aligned.** If you look in the mirror you will see that it is most likely your pelvis is tilted forward and, therefore, your whole upper body has followed, causing shortening of the leg muscles. We therefore need to practice altering the pelvis before we can alter the rest of the spine.

If you put your hands onto the front of your pelvis at the side, you will feel two bony points. These will be your reference points. They will probably be pointing down and forwards. You want to get them in a neutral position by tightening your tummy muscles and tucking your bottom in. The best way to do this is by *pelvic tilting* (see chapter 8). Once you have perfected this in the lying position, you can practice it sitting and standing.

When the pelvis is feeling more comfortable in its correct position (this will take weeks), you can then concentrate on the rest of the spine. Think of somebody pulling you up by a hair coming from the top of your head. Make sure your pelvis is positioned correctly and allow your spine to lift up; do not bend your knees. Hold this position and look in the mirror. Keep repeating and, once it begins to feel more normal, try walking in this position. The more you reinforce your posture, the quicker it will adapt. Good posture is not like the old army cartoons, with the chest and bottom sticking out; it is an 'S' shape alignment.

For you to achieve good posture, you must carry on with your exercises for strengthening, mobility and flexibility. Good posture is essential in the everyday activities of standing, lifting, sitting, and walking. If in doubt, think about your pelvic tilt and progress from there.

These exercises are essential parts of a pain management programme, and should be carried out every day.

chapter 5

RELAXATION TECHNIQUES FOR PAIN RELIEF

Relaxation techniques are so useful and safe that such techniques are often referred to as behavioural aspirin

Anonymous

What is meant by the *Relaxation Response*? What do we mean by the concept of *Deep Breathing*? What is meant by *Deep Muscle Relaxation* and *Progressive Muscle Relaxation*? What is *Autogenic Relaxation Training*? What is *Visualisation* and how does it act as an aid towards pain control? How often should relaxation be practiced to help reduce chronic pain?

If you are in pain you may become nervous about what is going to happen to you, especially if that pain has persisted for a long time. You may even wonder whether you are ever going to get rid of the pain, which for chronic pain sufferers is often present day and night. You are naturally anxious about when you will be able to resume your normal life-style, or return to work, if you have been in pain for a long time.

Not only are you anxious, but you may become depressed as well, and this is quite understandable. Your pulse rate increases, you constantly look worried (judging by your facial expression) and for some patients the whole personality may change. As was mentioned in chapter 3, when you are tense, pain is increased. Consequently, your pain tolerance falls and you become more sensitive to pain. Thus a continuous circle is set up. Pain leads to anxiety and depression, which reduce resistance to pain, producing more anxiety and depression. This may be referred to as the **"pain trap."**

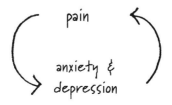

THE PAIN TRAP

Broken bones are placed in splints or plaster to aid rest. Migraine sufferers often report lying in a darkened room helps to abate an attack. An acutely inflamed joint or a strained or torn muscle demands rest until the episode is over and any swelling and spasm of the muscles has settled down. Similarly, the body as a whole also needs rest and sleep to recoup the strength it has lost due to the strain and tension of chronic pain.

If only you could relax, rest could be achieved more easily. Rest enables you to cope by breaking you free of the pain trap. Determining how much you will benefit from learning relaxation skills will very much depend on the type of personality you had prior to your pain. Some people are born worriers, others have an innate optimistic trait. Relaxation will not change your personality, but it will help you to cope with the pain of your illness.

If you are receptive to the benefits of relaxation therapy and understand the benefits of preventative daily usage, this form of therapy will enhance your overall pain management. Relaxation is a well-tried method of reducing or at least taking the edge off pain that is made worse by tension.

In summary, the art of learning relaxation seems to help to identify the effects of tension in three different ways:

- ☀ Pain is stressful and therefore increases levels of tension/anxiety.
- ☀ Pain increases guarded (hunched over, incorrect sitting) posture, which, over time, leads to increased pain.
- ☀ High levels of tension increase pain intensity ratings.

Relaxation also helps patients to gain extra feelings of control over their body. Feelings of well-being created by a patient help tension to disappear and, in turn, reduce pain. Research has also shown that relaxation significantly reduces blood pressure and muscle tension, and increases blood flow to the fingers and toes.

Relaxation therapy is widely used in medicine. Most of today's challenges require calm persistence or creative problem-solving. Both are easier to achieve when we are relaxed.

BREATHING STRESS AWAY

Proper breathing is an antidote to stress. We all breathe but few of us retain the habit of natural, deep breathing we have as infants. When you find muscle tension, nervous sweating, irregular breathing, or a rapid pulse because of pain, the best way to relax is to change the way you are breathing.

The lungs act as the carburettor of your body's engine. Correct slow deep breathing increases the oxygen level in your blood stream and sets the tone of many stress reactions in the body. Most people breathe from their middle chests in a somewhat rapid and shallow way when under stress. This may have evolved to help us accommodate short bursts of running or fighting, but is not a comfortable, long-term solution. Research also suggests that this can lead to high blood pressure.

DEEP BREATHING TECHNIQUE

Although this exercise can be practiced in a variety of poses, while first learning the technique the following is recommended:

- Lie on the floor in a warm room with a blanket or rug covering you. To aid concentration, turn on some relaxing music, dim the lights or close curtains or blinds. Bend your knees and move your feet about eight inches apart, with your toes turned slightly outwards. Make sure your spine is straight. It may help to lie on a sports mat.
- Scan your body for tension, become aware of what parts of your body are experiencing pain.
- Place one hand on your chest and one hand on your abdomen.
- Slowly begin to breathe in through your nose and count up to inhaling *one, two, three, four, five*. For best results, fill the abdome first, push it out and let it expand as far as you can, and as f

comfortable for you. After you fill the lower part of your lungs, let the chest rise up and out until the upper parts are filled. Leave about a second between each number.

☼ At the end of the count of five, your lungs should be nearly full. Slowly release (exhale) the air out through your mouth, counting backwards exhaling *five, four, three, two, one*. Make sure you empty your lungs almost entirely.

☼ To complete the exercise take two or three more of these deep, satisfying breaths.

People who are shallow breathers or cigarette smokers may feel a little light-headed after a lengthy deep-breathing exercise. This light-headedness comes from increased oxygen reaching the brain. Most of the time, the feeling is a comfortable, enjoyable sensation. Deep breathing naturally relaxes the body.

The beauty of this technique is that it can be used anywhere or during any activity. The next time you feel rushed or upset, breathe slowly and deeply. You can even do this exercise while you walk. Breathe in as you count four steps, out as you count the next four. Repeat as needed.

☼ Try to slow down in everything you do. Deep breathing will help you to do this. For example if your speech is fast or explosive, practice slowing down by using the deep breathing technique and notice the difference. If you eat quickly, slow down by taking slow deep breaths between chewing each piece of food.

☼ When you sit into your car, instead of automatically putting the key in the ignition and pulling across your safety belt, sit for 2 or 3 minutes and breathe slowly in and out. You can also do this while sitting in a traffic jam or waiting for the lights to change.

☼ The next time the phone rings, instead of grabbing the receiver, or running downstairs to answer it quickly, let it ring for a little longer and take one or two slow deep breaths. This will increase the relaxed state of the body and thus reduce risk of pain or spasms.

✻ When driving a car, you do not go from a neutral gear to ignoring first, second, third and fourth gear. Imagine th engine moving from neutral to top gear smoothly and, on __ __g~~~~, with the exhale, breathe slowly, returning to neutral. By using this image it may help you to enhance this simple, but hugely beneficial, relaxation skill. Any further techniques discussed in the chapter are all based on maximising the use of the deep breathing relaxation skill.

DEEP MUSCLE RELAXATION (DMR) AND PROGRESSIVE MUSCLE RELAXATION (PMR)

In 1938, Dr E Jacobson published a book, *Progressive Relaxation*, in which he described the use of *Deep Muscle Relaxation*. Dr Jacobson applied a simple biological principle to create a systematic method to relax the muscles of the body. To get a muscle to relax we must first tense, and then release it. Dr Jacobson developed a systematic series of tension release cycles to achieve relaxation. Research has shown that daily practice of such a technique can help the healing and management of several conditions such as ulcers, headaches, back pain and chronic pain.

Deep Muscle Relaxation is an excellent method to induce a calm state when ready to sleep, especially for patients with chronic pain. Some people when they become skilled at the technique even fall asleep at the end of the cycle. You can learn to sleep more soundly and consequently awaken fully rested.

PROGRESSIVE MUSCLE RELAXATION TECHNIQUE

Progressive relaxation is ideal for people who experience tensions in specific muscles. The nature of our lifestyles places us in certain positions (e.g. sitting, standing, walking, lying), all of which can generate tension. Sitting for long periods cuts down blood flow to the legs and can cause cramping and stiffness. An incorrect or uncomfortable sitting position can also cause back pain. Other common muscle tension complaints associated with chronic pain include low or middle back pain, stiff legs, neck stiffness, and chest/shoulder pain. All of these conditions can be relieved by correct and regular use of progressive muscle relaxation.

Further on is a list of general instructions that need to be understood before practising this technique. To begin with, you should practice at least once a day for 20-30 minutes. As you become skilled, you will need less time. Next, follow a general order of muscle groups to be relaxed. Begin with the hands and arms, then go to the head region, then down the body to the trunk, and finally to the legs and feet.

The progressive nature of the process will create a wave of relaxation flowing from muscle group to muscle group as you begin the tension release cycle. It is important that you focus your attention on the difference between a state of tension and a state of relaxation. In your mind compare the sensations and allow yourself to remember the feelings. Each tension release cycle consists of first tensing a specific muscle group and holding the muscles tensely for 10 seconds and then abruptly letting go. The best position to practice this technique is lying down or reclining into a chair to keep your body fully supported.

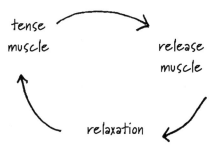

The exercises are listed below, and you can begin by practising in front of a mirror. It might be useful to put these exercises on tape to begin with.

RELAXING THE ARMS:

* Clench right hand (make a fist) and tense forearm - release.
* Repeat with left arm.
* Tense both right and left hands and forearms - release.
* Tense right biceps (front of upper arm) by bending right arm at elbow - release.
* Repeat with left arm.
* Tense right triceps (rear muscle upper arm) by stiffening right arm - release.
* Repeat with left arm.

RELAXING THE HEAD AREA:

* Wrinkle forehead - release.
* Raise your eyebrows as high as you can - release.
* Squeeze your eyelids tightly, but keep them closed without tension throughout the remainder of the exercises.
* Rotate eyes in a clockwise direction, returning to centre.
* Rotate eyes in an anticlockwise direction.
* Rotate your eyes to the right as far as you can.
* Rotate eyes to the left.
* Rotate eye to the top of the sockets.
* Rotate eye to the bottom of the eye sockets.
* Scrunch up your nose and cheeks - release.
* Purse your lips tightly together - release.
* Clench your jaws - release.
* Press your chin against your chest (as far as is comfortable for you) - release.
* Press tongue against the roof of your mouth - release.
* Begin to swallow, and hold - release. Tense throat - release.
* Tense throat and larynx muscles by humming a high note without

releasing any sound. Then hum back down the scale to the lowest note you can find.

RELAXING THE TRUNK:

☀ Tense shoulder muscles by raising your shoulders and touching your ears if you can - release.

☀ Pull shoulders back and tighten upper back muscles - release.

☀ Arch lower back and tighten low back muscles - release.

☀ Pull shoulders inward and tighten chest muscles - release.

☀ Tighten stomach muscles by pulling inward and downward - release.

☀ Tighten pelvic muscles in groin area - release.

☀ Pull in your buttocks and tighten them - release.

RELAXING THE LEGS:

☀ Tighten right upper leg - release.

☀ Tighten the left leg - release.

☀ Tense both upper legs - release.

☀ Pull legs together at knees and straighten legs - release.

☀ Tense right calf and shin (raise foot as though to touch leg) - release.

☀ Tense left calf and shin (raise foot as though to touch leg) - release.

☀ Tense right foot and toes - release.

☀ Tense left foot and toes - release.

ENHANCING RELAXATION THROUGHOUT THE BODY:

☀ Inhale slowly counting to 4, hold breath to a count of 4 and exhale slowly.

☀ Mentally scan the body for tension and maintain a state of slow deep breathing.

☀ Return to awakened aroused state by slowly getting up.

☀ Move your hands and arms, stretch if necessary.

☀ Move your feet and legs.

☀ Rotate your head slowly.

☀ Slowly open your eyes and sit up.

Some find it most beneficial to do these exercises first thing in the morning. Relaxing in the morning can be an excellent way to reduce the anticipatory tension/anxiety that chronic pain can bring throughout the day.

If you allow yourself to be creative, there are several ways you can apply progressive muscular relaxation. Remember you can do it completely or partially. So for example if your shoulders become tense and feel tight, you can go through the tension release for this muscle group only. You can even indulge in this limited application while performing tasks such as walking or writing.

*A*UTOGENIC RELAXATION

Autogenic relaxation is a form of self-hypnosis. *Autogenic* means applying a technique to yourself by yourself. The format is simple and involves repeating a series of self-instructions (e.g. *"My arms are warm"*) several times while you experience and observe such sensations as described by the instructions. You only have to observe, there should be no effort to make it happen.

In fact, research has shown that if you try too hard to make something happen, the opposite often occurs. This type of technique encourages us to give up control in order to exercise control. The rules for practising autogenic relaxation are similar to those for other methods.

- Assume a comfortable position in which the body is not strained and is well-supported. Loosen any tight clothing or jewellery. Dim the lights in a quiet atmosphere. You must be prepared to mentally observe the sensations in your body with the instruction.
- Deep breathing will help to enhance the relaxed state. End each session with some movements of the body to re-establish a state of alertness, and with a positive affirmation (e.g. "When I open my eyes, I will feel relaxed and refreshed ready to face the day ahead.").

INSTRUCTIONS FOR AUTOGENIC RELAXATION

Say to yourself:

- ❋ My hands and arms are relaxed, heavy and warm (5 times).
- ❋ My feet and legs are relaxed, heavy and warm (5 times).
- ❋ My abdomen is relaxed, warm and comfortable (5 times).
- ❋ My breathing is slow, deep and even (10 times).
- ❋ My pulse is relaxed, calm and regular (10 times).
- ❋ My forehead is relaxed and cool (5 times).
- ❋ When I open my eyes, I will feel relaxed and ready to face the day.
- ❋ Move hands and arms, feet and legs. Rotate head. Sit up slowly.

Because the autogenic relaxation process is simple and internal, you can practice it while performing tasks. Many find it useful to help prepare for sleep. Although you will achieve greater relaxation with your eyes closed, you can also practice this technique with your eyes open. Therefore, you can even practice while standing in a bus queue without anybody being the wiser.

VISUALISATION

You can reduce stress significantly using the imagination. The practice of positive thinking in the treatment of physical symptoms was popularised by *Emil Coué*, a French pharmacist, at the turn of the century. He believed that the power of the imagination far exceeds that of the will. It is difficult to will yourself into a relaxed state, but you can *imagine* relaxation spreading through your body, and you can *visualise* yourself in a safe and beautiful retreat.

Coué asserted that all of your thoughts become reality. For example if you think sad thoughts, you feel unhappy. In order to release your body of pain, you can refocus your mind on positive healing images.

Visualisation is practiced and studied in cancer and pain centres throughout the world. Stephanie Matthews and O. Carl Simonton, who pioneered the use of visualisation with cancer patients, wrote *Getting Well* in 1980.

Because patients know that switching attention from the pain helps them to notice it less, professionals have developed methods to help sufferers attention-switch, or reinterpret the sensation. For example, imagining a sudden pain as a heavy or massage-like pressure reduces the fear of the pain and the patient feels more in control.

Another method of using visualisation is to learn to switch attention away from the site of pain and to build up a scene in your mind (e.g. a deep wood, by a river, by the sea, in a country cottage) and imagine yourself there. This takes you right out of the present and into a newly-created, pain-free place.

Research has shown that this reinterpretation method seems to work best. The process of using imagery to relax is simple: Assume a comfortable position, close your eyes, and create an image in your mind of some place where you feel truly relaxed, calm and happy. In this picture, observe what is happening around you. Notice sounds, colours and smell. Become aware of movement, familiar objects, and notice the freshness of the air. Let yourself become aware of positive feelings. Breathe slowly, deeply, and relax.

Most of us use visualisation in our daily lives, but few of us consciously use this process to relax. Visualisation can be used as an efficient method to relax and create a positive frame of mind. It is quick, and it can be used easily in the most difficult of situations to help lessen and manage pain.

HOW TO GET THE MOST FROM USING RELAXATION

A basic premise of this chapter is that the benefits of relaxation techniques can only be fully realised after they have been practiced regularly over a period of time. Intellectual understanding of most techniques is of little value, unless accompanied by first-hand experience. Most pain management programmes will provide the opportunity to help develop personal familiarity with them.

The length of time required each day to practice relaxation techniques varies. It is best to spend some time doing the exercises of your choice every day. If seven days a week seems too much, plan shorter relaxation periods to be incorporated into your daily structure or routine. Do not expect them to just happen: plan carefully in advance and choose a quiet place where you will be uninterrupted. Since this is a new activity for most people living with chronic pain, it is wise to explain to the people around you what you are doing. Ask them to help you by giving you privacy without any distractions. Family members, fellow workers and friends tend to be very supportive once they understand what you are doing and why.

The purpose of regular practice is twofold. Firstly, it will ensure that you will be able to carry out the exercises consciously anytime you need to, without having to refer to written materials or tapes. Secondly, regular practice will develop the habit of relaxing at an unconscious level. If for some reason you are unable to do your exercises one day, treat this as if you have missed an appointment with a busy professional. Give yourself the same courtesy as you would a missed appointment: reschedule! This means you start again tomorrow.

If you are not a very highly motivated person or have a history of poor self-discipline, seek the help of a family member or friend that will agree to practice with you. In this way you can share your experiences, support and encouragement.

Tell your doctor that you intend to practice relaxation techniques, and discuss whether your physical symptoms are exacerbated by stress/anxiety, or if there are specific physiological causes as well. Once you start, consult your doctor if you are still experiencing prolonged physical ill-effects.

chapter 6

THE ROLE OF COMPLEMENTARY THERAPIES IN PAIN MANAGEMENT

Complementary therapies have become much more accepted over the last decade. Many GPs now prescribe complementary treatments in conjunction with conventional medicine and sometimes they are recommended as the preferred treatment. In Britain over 40% of GPs offer complementary medicine within their practices and many more refer their patients to alternative practitioners.

Both complementary and conventional medicines have their place in the management of the chronic pain sufferer. With some conditions modern drugs and surgery are necessary. Many turn to complementary therapies when they feel that they have run out of solutions from the conventional networks. In the case of the chronic pain sufferer there may be many symptoms secondary to the initial complaints e.g. depression, stress, muscle tension or stomach ulcers. In many of these cases complementary therapy combined with the more conventional methods of treatment can be beneficial.

The scientific basis of many of the therapies mentioned here has not been established. Opinion is divided about the value of some of them, and it is essential to appreciate that claims made by complementary practitioners *can* be false. Before embarking on a course of complementary therapy consult with your doctor or physiotherapist to ensure there are no contra-indications. Always use a qualified practitioner (see addresses at the end of book) and never self-diagnose. If you attend complementary therapists, make sure they know your history and details of any medication you may be taking.

PHYSIOTHERAPY

Though not categorised as a complementary therapy, physiotherapy does complement conventional treatments and is often the treatment of choice by doctors. Physiotherapists are qualified to deal with musculoskeletal elements of the chronic pain sufferer and are able to give advice on the ergonomic and functional difficulties to be overcome when suffering from pain.

If you are referred to a physiotherapist in the early stages of rehabilitation they will be concerned with the reduction of any inflammation in the joints and muscles, and with mobilising the affected areas. To this end, they may use electrotherapy such as *interferential* and *ultrasound*,: hot or cold treatments which will help to speed up the healing process by increasing the blood supply and removing the toxins. Hot and cold treatments have the benefit of reducing muscle spasms and can be used safely at home. A hot bath or a hot water bottle wrapped in a towel can work wonders on a tense muscle group.

Recently available are *heat packs*, which can be warmed in a microwave oven and used directly. Cold packs are best used on a more acute lesion, like a pulled muscle. A packet of frozen peas wrapped in 3 layers of wet towel can be very effective applied to the area for 10 minutes. If you feel any burning on the area you must remove the ice immediately, as it can damage the skin. If your sensation is defective, the same warning applies to heat application. If in doubt, do not use it.

Physiotherapists may use manual manipulation or mobilisation to encourage movement of joints and tissues. There are many different techniques used, the object being to gain an increased range of movement. You will be given a course of exercises to continue at home, which will maintain and improve muscle movement and help to develop some muscle strength.

You may be referred to your physiotherapist for *traction* if you have developed some peripheral pain due to injury. Traction utilises a special couch with a head halter for the neck or a pelvic belt for the lower back. The therapist will position you, allowing the affected joint to be stretched. The theory is that the joints are freed from the pressure of the muscle spasm and allow release of tissues and realignment of the joints which may have been pressing on a nerve.

Not all peripheral pain responds to traction and your physiotherapist will determine if this is the most appropriate form of treatment.

If you attend a physiotherapist in the more chronic stages of your rehabilitation, you will be assessed thoroughly to judge how your body has responded to being in long-term chronic pain. Your posture, range of movement, muscle power, gait patterns, pain levels, flexibility and co-ordination will also be assessed followed by treatment of specific areas requiring attention - joint stiffness or muscle tightness. But the main aim is to help you to help yourself by carrying out a series of strengthening, stretching and mobilising exercises within your ability. Posture and correct ergonomics in the workplace and at home will be discussed. In short, you will be taught how best to manage your pain and prevent further injury.

The physiotherapist you attend should be chartered.

ACUPUNCTURE

Acupuncture, derived from the Latin word *acus* meaning *needle,* is a method of puncturing or pricking. Acupuncture has been practiced in China for about 5,000 years. The archeological discovery of flint, bamboo and bone needles suggests that acupuncture existed long before the discovery of metal. In the 17th century, doctors introduced acupuncture to Europe but it did not become popular until the 1970s.

One of the best known and widely used of the Eastern therapies, it is a useful tool in achieving pain relief in many conditions, from arthritis and muscle disorders to childbirth. It is based on the Chinese theory that the body consists of two opposing forces, *Yin* and *Yang*. The balance of these two forces is essential for well-being. If the balance is disturbed, the result can be illness or pain. The interaction of the two forces gives rise to *chi,* the life-energy that flows through 12 *meridians* or channels around the body. Acupuncturists believe that an even flow of *chi* through these pathways is essential for health. There are 365 *acupoints* along these meridians at which *chi* is concentrated and through which it enters and leaves the body. It is thought that illness is caused by an obstruction of this energy. An acupuncturist will make a diagnosis by taking a full history, noting your appearance, colour and smell. The checking of all 12 meridian pulses will tell him/her about imbalances in your body.

Acupuncture treatment consists of having several very fine needles, which are made from stainless steel tipped with copper, inserted into different parts of the body for a period of 30 to 90 minutes. A course of 10-12 sessions is usually recommended.

Sometimes dried *mugwort* (or *moxa*) is burned to generate heat on the acupoint for some conditions such as low back pain. Your pulses are checked after treatment to ensure that it has been effective. You may feel tired afterwards and the pain may worsen before getting better.

Acupuncture has five medically understandable effects:

1 The 'fight or flight' response that occurs when the skin is punctured will bring a relief of pain.

2 An analgesic effect is caused when the skin is punctured and endorphins are secreted.

3 Sensory impulses from the skin will block impulses from the pain-carrying nerves - the same principle as when you press on a toothache and the pain is relieved.

4 Muscle relaxation is produced by the bombardment of impulses from trigger points. This, in turn, helps to reduce pain.

5 Stress reduction is achieved by the relaxed atmosphere, and a feeling that you are doing something active towards managing your pain: "A problem shared is a problem halved."

It must be added that, in general, Western medical practitioners do not subscribe to an unqualified acceptance of this theory. Western medicine suggests acupuncture acts as a blocking of pain messages as in the 'gate' control theory and the raising of endorphin levels as discussed in chapter 1.

A qualified practitioner should be considered for this treatment

ALEXANDER TECHNIQUE

Frederick Mathias Alexander was born in Tasmania, Australia in 1869. He was a Shakespearean actor who suffered from constant sore throats, which led to loss of voice and hoarseness. He developed the *Alexander Technique* as an alternative to rest and medication which gave him only temporary relief. He felt that something in his lifestyle was causing the problem. He developed the technique by observing himself closely for many years. He used a mirror to study particular movements and discovered that over the years his body had picked up many bad habits which were inhibiting the body's natural functions. For example, he noted that when he spoke he pulled his head back which caused a depression of his larynx and therefore an increase in pressure of the vocal chords which was causing his problem.

The Alexander Technique aims to re-educate the body so that it is properly used in its most natural way. The basic principle is that correct use helps function; poor use inhibits it. Our physical well-being is affected by misuse of our bodies; muscles, joints, circulation, respiration, lymphatic and nervous systems are all tainted to some degree. This, in turn, causes problems with the mechanics of the body and postural deviation, which can give rise to pain in many areas. The Alexander Technique aims to help induce the good habits which will aid both physical and mental well-being. The technique is taught individually to clients by trained teachers.

The number of lessons required depends on the degrees of disability and the client's willingness to adapt. During the lessons the teacher will move and guide the parts of the body into their natural position and instruct the student to do the same.

This is not a technique in which you carry out a specific programme; the learned movements must be used in all aspects of your daily routine from opening a door to drinking a cup of tea. It encourages more fluidity of movement and an improvement in posture which will help to reduce stress on individual parts of the body and aid the reduction of pain. The great advantage of this technique is that it is very gentle and therefore useful for many ages and degrees of disability.

AROMATHERAPY

Herbal oils have been used for many centuries to treat illness and promote well being. *Aromatherapy* is a treatment by the application of pure essential oils. Essential oils were developed in Persia about 1,000 years ago, and were brought to Europe by the crusaders. The oils are extracted from the leaves, stems and flowers of plants. The usual method of obtaining the oils is by subjecting the plant to heat, steam or boiling. Aromatherapy as we know it today is based largely on research by French doctors.

The oils are used by inhalation in the following ways:

- By adding drops to a bath.
- By adding drops to a bowl of water and placing on a gentle heat (e.g. radiator).
- By using an oil burner.
- By massage.

The principle behind aromatherapy is that the nervous system is influenced by the oil molecules entering through the bloodstream. This assists both the physical and emotional well-being. The oils will help to achieve a balance in these systems, and so aid the healing process. This process is disputed by conventional medical practitioners who claim the effect is purely one of relaxation, but this is also beneficial.

Many essential oils can be bought from chemists and health food shops. Always follow instructions for dilution and check if there are any contraindications for the oil you are using.

ELECTROTHERAPY

If you are attending a physiotherapist, electrical therapy may be recommended as part of your treatment. The most common forms are *ultrasound, interferential* and *short wave diathermy*. These treatments can temporarily reduce pain but will not help the underlying problem. A physiotherapist or doctor may provide you with or advise you to try a *TENS machine*. This is a version of the acupuncture principle of pain-blocking (see chapter 1 for *Gate Theory*). If the touch fibres on the skin are stimulated, the pain messages passing into the spinal cord are blocked. Each TENS machine has small pads which are coated with a jelly to ensure contact with the skin. These are placed over the body's trigger points and stimulated by a low frequency current, which produces a tingling sensation which is not painful. The feeling should be that of a 'good' pain, with the original pain being diminished and overridden by the tingling.

TENS is most effective if you have only one or two painful areas. Because the machines are equipped with a limited number of pads, usually 2-4, only a small number of areas can be treated simultaneously.

Finding the most effective use of the TENS machines is by trial and error, placing the electrodes on different trigger spots and experimenting with different intensities. They are a useful self-help tool, especially in reducing muscle spasm/pain, and many patients use them regularly. You should be taught how to use a machine by a qualified practitioner for electrode placement and operating frequencies. You may find that you need help in attaching the pads, especially if you have middle back pain.

The TENS is safe if used correctly and there is no danger of electrocution if your machine is made by a reputable company. TENS machines should not be used if you have a cardiac pacemaker or are pregnant, and should never be placed on the front of the neck or near the eyes. An allergic reaction to the rubber pads is a possibility.

FELDENKRAS

The *Feldenkras Technique* was developed by Dr Moshe Feldenkras. Its aim is to improve posture, mobility and general health by increasing awareness through movement. Feldenkras began his career as an engineer and physicist. He was a keen sportsman, and an injury to his knee prompted him to study human mechanics in great depth.

The technique consists of teaching a series of exercises and principles. Feldenkras feels that the mind and the body are inextricably linked, and that the state of mind will be reflected in muscle tone and posture. Similarly, he believes that if body patterns are changed, for example due to an accident, they can affect the mental well-being of a person.

The initial exercises are taught lying on the floor, and then progressed into sitting and standing postures. All exercises are done slowly and should cause very little discomfort.

Many physiotherapists are Feldenkras trained, and they integrate these techniques with the more standard exercise programmes.

HOMEOPATHY

A physician called *Samuel Hahnemann* (1755-1843) started this therapy in Germany. Primitive treatments during his era, such as the cutting of veins to release unhealthy blood, were carried out regularly. The mortality rate from these treatments was very high and patients would probably have recovered without them.

Hahnemann felt that when a drug or treatment was given to suppress a disease or symptom that the illness would manifest itself in some other form. In *homeopathy* a substance is given that will produce the symptoms of the disease but, as these are given in minute quantities, they will stimulate the body's own repair mechanisms.

The remedies used in homeopathy were developed by administering the substances to a healthy body and observing their effects. There is a similarity between modern day vaccination and homeopathy in that a vaccination introduces a mild form of a disease into the system; the body will then form antibodies to the disease itself. Some GPs, as well as natural medicine practitioners, are now using homeopathy. To treat the patient, the homeopath must take a very detailed history including lifestyle, diet and pain patterns. The compilation of symptoms will help diagnose the disease and how the patient will respond.

Homeopathy is not an obvious choice of treatment for the chronic pain sufferer as it is very difficult to reproduce pain in a particular area using a remedy, but there are specific homeopathic remedies for a large number of conditions, many of which may be responsible for chronic pain (e.g. a prolapsed disc). There is also a homeopathic anti-inflammatory drug widely used by practitioners. Your GP may suggest some homeopathic remedies as opposed to the traditional pain-killers and anti-inflammatories, especially if you have stomach problems.

HYDROTHERAPY

We have already outlined the benefits of exercising in water. A series of exercises in a heated pool is very beneficial for someone in pain as the body is supported in the water and does not have to rely on the muscles and joints to keep the body in the upright position. With the body supported, it is easier to gain maximum movement of joints and muscles with minimum strain. The use of floats is beneficial, allowing a particularly painful area to be supported whilst another is exercised. Floats can also be used to allow total relaxation of the body. If you are strengthening a particular group of muscles, floats can be used as a resistance in the water.

Hydrotherapy classes run by a physiotherapist are the most beneficial, as exercises can be tailored specifically to the individual's needs. Once you have mastered these, you can continue them unsupervised. Many patients find relief in Jacuzzis and spas, often finding the jets of water combined with the heat help to reduce muscle spasm. Exercise in water with intermittent rests in the Jacuzzi seems to be particularly beneficial. This gives only temporary relief, but is useful as part of a comprehensive programme.

The most accessible hydrotherapy of all is of course a hot bath or shower. Add some aromatherapy oils to the bath to aid relaxation. Some people have difficulty getting in and out of the bath: the only alternative is allowing a hot shower to run on the painful area for a length of time. Put a plastic chair or stool in the shower cubicle if you have difficulty in standing for long periods.

MASSAGE

There are many different types of massage available and the array of choices can be confusing. Massage has been developed from the basic human instinct of rubbing or stroking a painful area. Massage itself will not cure the underlying problem but it will certainly help to relax the body and mind, thereby relieving pain and tension. The therapeutic effects of massage are to improve the lymphatic system circulation and aid the elimination of impurities. This will increase the body's healing power and increase relaxation and flexibility of muscles. Massage can be administered at home if you have a friend or partner who is a willing helper; often used in conjunction with aromatherapy oils it can help reduce tension especially in the neck area.

Some of the types of massage are:
- **Swedish massage:** a set pattern of strokes designed to improve circulation and muscle tone.
- **Ki Massage:** traditional massage techniques combined with healing designed to work in conjunction with the person's energy (chi).
- **Deep tissue massage/rolling massage and mild manipulation:** to improve mobility of muscles and joints in conjunction with exercises to improve posture.
- **Remedial massage:** to improve flexibility of muscles and joints in conjunction with an exercise programme.

MEDICAL HERBALISM

This is probably the oldest form of medical treatment but the use of herbs in their natural form has been curtailed by the growth of the pharmaceutical industry, which continues to draw largely on these natural sources e.g. *digitalis* from the foxglove and *morphine* from the poppy. The main reason that synthetic drugs are preferred to the raw form is that the exact dosage can be calculated whereas in the raw form the potency varies from plant to plant.

Herbalists treat the whole body and may work in combination with other alternative practitioners e.g. an osteopath who in the case of the chronic pain sufferer may manipulate an affected area whilst the herbalist prescribes a poultice or ointment to ease muscle tenderness.

Herbs, as with any medication, should be taken only under supervision of a qualified herbalist. Just because they are herbs does not mean they are without dangers and side-effects.

MEDITATION

Meditation is very beneficial in reducing stress, inducing relaxation and taking the focus away from pain. The great advantage of meditation is that it can be done anywhere at any time once the basic techniques have been acquired. Meditation is often an integral part of complementary treatments such as *Yoga* and *T'ai Chi*.

One of the most popular types is *Transcendental Meditation*. This involves sitting comfortably in a secure environment with the eyes closed. A *mantra*, (an easily remembered and repeatable sound) is repeated. This mantra will be given to you by your instructor.

Thoughts will enter and leave the mind and eventually the mantra will be at the forefront. The mind will then become peaceful allowing the body to relax. The practice starts under supervision, and once mastered the technique can be used at home. It is very important to have time out when you suffer from chronic pain, and this is a good way to achieve that.

OSTEOPATHY

Osteopathy originated in America in the late 19th century. It was created by Andrew Suil, who felt that any structural problems in the body would interfere with the nerve or blood supply and prevent healing. As mechanical problems are often a cause of chronic pain, osteopathy may prove beneficial.

The treatment usually involves gentle manipulation of the body's skeletal system. This is believed to release areas of pressure, which will help to improve blood circulation and lymphatic flow, which will in turn stimulate the body's natural healing mechanisms.

As with all complementary therapies, if you find your condition deteriorating, discuss with your doctor.

REFLEXOLOGY

The first record of reflexology was found in Egypt in about 2300 BC. It was not until 1913 that it re-emerged in the United States as a treatment. A masseuse called Eunice Ingham worked in conjunction with a Dr Riley researching and experimenting with pressure massage to the feet.

Modern day reflexology divides the body into 10 vertical and 3 horizontal zones. The foot is also divided into 10 vertical and 3 horizontal zones. The zones of the feet relate to the zones of the body eg the zone for the heart is on the left foot, the big toe relates to the head.

By massaging and manipulating the feet, a reflexologist can determine if there are any blockages in the zones. The therapist will take a patient history and visually assess the foot, giving a diagnostic picture.

Any 'blockages' found in the foot will be broken down by a massage technique to allow the energy to flow freely. The length of a session varies according to the number of blockages, size of feet and the patient's tolerance.

Reflexology would not be of specific use in reducing the cause of chronic pain, but it may relieve conditions associated with it such as insomnia, stress, headaches or poor circulation.

SHIATSU

Shiatsu means finger pressure. Developed in Japan, it has its roots in the same oriental tradition as acupuncture. Shiatsu techniques include stretching, holding and leaning body weight into various parts of the patient's anatomy to improve energy flow, blood circulation, flexibility and posture.

Pressure is applied through the hands, thumbs, fingers, forearms, knees and feet. The purpose of this pressure is to balance and harmonise the *chi* energy in the body in a similar manner to acupuncture.

In general, a shiatsu treatment will cover the whole body but, occasionally, the practitioner will work on a specific area if there appears to be an energy blockage in a particular meridian.

Shiatsu claims to be effective in the treatment of most illnesses including sinusitis, depression, arthritis and back pain. Therapists state that most illnesses have both a physical and emotional cause. They diagnose the physical, emotional and spiritual blockages and will attempt an energy rebalance by a process of unblocking.

Each application of Shiatsu pressure is a diagnosis allowing the therapist to treat the body's condition. The hands and the fingers detect abnormalities in the skin or muscles, and determine irregularities.

The positive aspects of Shiatsu therapy is that there are no side-effects and that it is a suitable treatment for any age group and degree of disability.

AI CHI

a generalised form of exercise and meditative therapy, which ,ed in China in the 11th century. The aim of *T'ai Chi* is to strengthen and invigorate the entire person by carrying out a set of very exact movements which require a great deal of concentration. Each movement requires a degree of strength, flexibility, co-ordination and concentration. An important facet of these exercises is breathing control which is very important in the chronic pain sufferer, as stress, tension and pain lead to shallow and ineffective breathing.

Pain management groups have enjoyed and benefited from T'ai Chi classes. In fact, many of them choose to continue with this form of exercise on completion of the course. The exercises are difficult at the outset due to the combination of skills needed to complete them, but under supervision, they are taught very gradually and progressed slowly, allowing an advance when a set of exercises has been mastered. The benefit of T'ai Chi is that it combines mental relaxation with physical exercise without over-exertion.

YOGA

Yoga has become a very popular form of exercise and relaxation over recent years in the Western world. It is most certainly a useful exercise for chronic pain sufferers.

The yoga method of exercise is a combination of gentle exercise, stretching and relaxation designed to enhance the life force of the body. The different types of Yoga have different emphases. *Hatha Yoga*, for example, concentrates on posture, which is useful if you need to increase muscle strength and flexibility, whereas *Raja Yoga* focus on mental control which is helpful if stress is playing a part in chronic pain. Yoga will not cure the underlying cause, but will help with improving mental outlook and increasing physical strength, fitness and flexibility.

Always ensure that a teacher is aware of any physical problems before you commence a class; good teachers will take a history before they start. Many of the exercises will be manageable, but there may be some which will exacerbate problems. In this case, abstain or under the guidance of your teacher progress very slowly. Relaxation of the mind as well as the body is one of the great benefits of participating in a Yoga class.

chapter 7

SELF-HELP IN
PAIN MANAGEMENT

What are the key features of the person who learns to live with chronic pain? What is meant by the concept of *self-help* in pain management? How can you learn to play an active role in your own recovery from a physical and psychological perspective? How can you combine the advice you receive from your medical practitioner, psychologist and physiotherapist?

Throughout these chapters you have been given a detailed knowledge of the definitions of chronic pain with emphasis on the idea that the true onus is on *you*, the sufferer or patient, to bring about change in your life. Change comes from within and it is essential to make the decision to stop searching for the cure: take charge of your life and begin living with chronic pain.

You have been given advice on the importance of regular and safe exercise routines, the most appropriate medical intervention to seek out, and how to learn the skills of effective relaxation. Our beliefs regarding the possible benefits of some complementary therapies have also been shared with you.

We have tried to keep the book as jargon-free as possible to enable everyone to benefit from our experience and skills.

The following is a list of guidelines for self-help in pain management.

TEN KEY ELEMENTS OF PAIN MANAGEMENT

1.   Learn to live

For many months, even years, several patients with chronic pain have stopped living their lives. Essentially the pain they live with has put them on hold. As professionals working in the area of pain management, we see this every day in our practice. Freud in *'Civilisation And Its Discontents'* explains this in detail; he refers to it as *thanatos* or the *death wish* (*thanatos* is the Greek for death). The decision to learn to live again is not so easy for many people.

Step 1

Ask yourself: "Do I want to learn to live with my pain?" If you did not hesitate to answer "Yes" then continue on to Step 2.

Step 2

Keep asking yourself the question: "Do I want to learn to live again?" until you are absolutely sure that you can make an affirmative decision.

Step 3

Arriving here means you have made the decision and are ready to learn to live a new life managing your pain. If you have reached Step 3, then you have created the foundation for resistance to chronic pain.

Only then can you commit yourself to your work, family, and to life. Emotional engagement is paramount towards self-help in pain management.

2.   Develop Positive Reasons for Living

Once you develop positive reasons for living, what will emerge are specific goals to work towards, both at a physical and psychological level. You can continuously update old goals and create new ones: whatever works best for you. When a goal is achieved it is important to move on and create a new challenge. Once we have goals for living, these will provide motivation for striving. Goals serve as benchmarks, and will not only enhance the patient's well-being but also the welfare of those around them. Life without goals and an ability to pace ourselves towards these goals can lead to self-destruction and detract from self-respect and well-being.

Write a list of your goals and review it at least once a day. Display it in a location where it is clearly visible to you as you go about your daily activities. When the vicissitudes of life create unbearable pressure and perhaps increase your pain intensity, pull out your list and remind yourself of goals already achieved.

3. Decide how to live

Once people decide to live and persevere with chronic pain they can then formulate how they will live within acceptable and safe physical and mental limits. Motivated patients will want more than just survival; they will want to thrive. Once you decide you want to live life as fully as possible, you will have to create that sense of well-being in many different dimensions.

The following are specific areas that you can influence:

☀ The body

Set guidelines for healthy eating and maintaining a correct body weight. Check your ideal body weight with your doctor or dietician.

Select the ideal number of hours of sleep you require. If your sleep is broken, relaxation exercises will help get the deepest sleep possible. Restful sleep is healing and regenerating.

Set a goal to experience pleasure from your body - complementary therapy, swimming, or increasing overall fitness by means of an exercise programme.

☀ Work

Work is important for financial reasons and for allowing us to use skills or to relearn and update them.

Sometimes career choices or occupational roles may change due to injuries and chronic pain. Write down the necessary steps in pursuing this path or seek the advice of a career consultant who has experience in rehabilitation.

Retirement may be inevitable for many patients. Can you perhaps afford to work on a part-time basis if this best suits your pain threshold?

☼ Family

In some pain management programmes the family is brought in for a *Family Day*. Chronic pain patients often lose intimacy in their lives and it is important that the pain management team addresses this with each patient in turn. Family members benefit greatly from using such a forum to voice their frustrations and tensions in living with a chronic pain sufferer. Often this is the only opportunity they get to open up, and speak their minds without fear of offending the sufferer. Encouragement and the creation of a safe and confidential environment is of paramount importance at this meeting.

☼ Independence

Independence is often something patients say they have lost as a result of their pain. Patients should be encouraged to develop an acceptable degree of independence. This does not mean isolation or a license to create loneliness within family life. After all many patients have made the decision to live a better life with chronic pain because of their families or loved one.

☼ Emotions

Set goals for openly expressing your feelings. Let yourself experience and express your anger, sadness, fear, disappointment and joy. Suppression of feelings leads to tension in the body which can lead to increased pain.

☼ Relaxation time

Schedule relaxation time around your family routines. Set up a regular pattern for practice. Research suggests that daily relaxation leads to fewer sick days and less illness. Ask your family to support the need to create a quiet atmosphere in the home when you are trying to relax.

4. Think positive and develop an optimistic attitude

Even in the face of adversity, patients with a positive attitude expect success because they are confident in their own abilities. To view life's vicissitudes as challenges you need an optimistic attitude. This attitude has certain core beliefs that people review mentally to maintain a positive attitude.

Examples of affirmations include:

> ☀ *Life works out for the best.*
> ☀ *I can learn from my experience of pain.*
> ☀ *I can make things turn out well for me.*
> ☀ *Every day in every way I am getting better and better.*

P.M.A. (**P**ositive **M**ental **A**ttitude) will change your way of thinking about pain. We suggest patients take a daily attitude check.

- ☀ Record your pattern of negative thinking on a daily basis.
- ☀ Ask yourself what you can do to change such negative thinking patterns.
- ☀ Replace each negative thought with a positive thought.
- ☀ Compliment and reward yourself for positive thinking.

5. Take control of your life

The chronic pain patient must learn to become a master of their fate. Pain management teaches patients to be in control of their lives. Before learning pain management skills, patients typically view themselves as helpless victims. As you have already learned from previous chapters, out of that perceived helplessness, they experience anxiety and depression. Depression puts life on hold.

Frequently, chronic pain patients carry on internal dialogues that emphasise their feelings of powerlessness and loss of control. By making such statements as "I just cannot take any more pain," or "The pain has me at the end of my rope" reveal that such patients are consumed by stress and pressure. What is required is to change a **negative** cognitive style into a **positive** cognitive style (*cognitive* meaning our perception). With this in mind the internal dialogue then becomes "The pain is rough, but I can take charge of it" or "The pain will pass and I'll be fine." The change in statements shows that a recognition of 'feeling in control' acts as a very powerful weapon against pain. Such an attitude can be learned with the help of the pain management team.

Changing the way we use language also helps to take control of the way you think. If you say "I cannot do x," change it to "I am choosing not to do x." Such a change in thinking hands the onus back to the patient. It might also help to keep a diary of feelings, thoughts and events surrounding your pain. You can then discuss your thoughts and feelings with the psychologist. Assess how such thoughts and feelings change as you learn to take control of your life. Try to de-sensitise yourself to negative thoughts and feelings. Practice what is commonly referred to as *The Self-Control Dialogue*. A pain management programme may include a *no-pain day*, during which patients try for one day not to discuss their pain with group members and families. Notice how hard it is to stop talking about your pain.

6. Be open to learning

The patient in chronic pain must try to operate in an open learning mode. In other words, they must try to develop divergent thinking patterns and be creative. Divergent thinking occurs when a person considers many different alternatives in the appraisal of a situation that triggers pain. This thinking increases a patient's self-confidence. Convergent thinking on the other hand means a person sees few alternatives and options. They lose the ability to think creatively, and this kind of thinking and helplessness are core characteristics of people suffering from depression.

The first rule in developing an attitude where you are open to learning means that you must stop trying to prove yourself. Secondly you must view errors or failures as opportunities. The third step is to try to develop a learning dialogue. In other words practice statements such as:

  ☀ *What can I learn from my experience of pain?*
  ☀ *What benefits are there from trying to manage my pain?*
  ☀ *This pain provides me with a chance to slow down and learn new life-skills.*

Patients often look confused during the first week of a pain management course when the psychologist asks them if they can see any advantages to their pain. As the weeks progress, they add daily to their list of advantages and move from convergent to divergent thinking skills.

7. View each opportunity for change as a challenge

The skills taught on any pain management programme try to instruct a patient to view each situation regarding their pain as an opportunity to learn, to grow and to enrich their lives. Thrivers who participate in a pain management programme *believe* that they will overcome an obstacle and will benefit in the process of tackling the challenge. This is especially true when patients are encouraged to structure their day around the skills the pain management team have taught them.

Awareness is the first step towards challenge. Observe your thinking when the doctor, psychologist or physiotherapist requests you to do something you have not done in a while. Question the benefits of the situation. Apply such questions to every area of your life. Develop the 'What's in it for me' syndrome and you will soon leave your tension and anxiety behind you.

When structuring your day, be realistic and slowly increase your goals - do not take on too much at once.

8. Become a problem-solver

Negative thoughts focus on failure, loss and the expectation of a negative outcome. Each problem regarding pain must be clearly defined both from a physical and mental point of view. Once such definitions are formed, each task can be taken on board and the patient can work towards an acceptable solution. The process of worrying about pain is a psychological defence. Worrying creates more tension and reinforces what we referred to earlier as the *'pain trap.'*

Problem-solving works in the following way:

☀ By stepping back and gaining a perspective.

☀ By looking at your predicament.

☀ By asking yourself questions like "What is the roadblock in my depression?" "Am I paying too much attention to my pain?"

Create an objective and ask questions like "What do I hope to achieve from my life?" "What do I want to accomplish now within my new physical limitations?" Ask yourself "What are the best solutions?" This involves a high level of compromise because you have to stop living in the past and comparing the way you lived before chronic pain to your present situation.

Do not always expect to find the solution on your own, discuss it not only with professionals, but also with family, friends and work colleagues.

9. Become an active participant

Many people with chronic pain tend to be passive in their attitudes and behaviours. Resiliency involves accepting your feelings and thoughts, whatever they may be, and then actively changing what you do not want to experience. An active participant uses change to their advantage, and this is hugely important in learning effective pain management skills.

Some professionals as well as patients struggle with the reality that you, the patient, are responsible for your fate, health, thinking, feeling and behaviour.

Equally true responsibility involves accepting feedback both positive and negative. For example, during one of our family days a patient was very disappointed, as she had believed that her progress was excellent, where her partner said he saw no difference in her. When this was later discussed it was discovered that this lady's partner was comparing her activity levels to the time prior to her injuries and not to when she started pain management. Recognition of this was positive for both, and progress for everyone was maintained.

Active, responsible chronic pain sufferers believe in themselves, have high self-confidence and will consistently strive to improve. Active participation in your own recovery process not only enhances your pain state but your future resistance to disease and stress. The matrix of active involvement in pain management allows you to strive without being driven. It moves beyond the traditional medical model of treatment and treats the whole person with an enhanced likelihood of physical and mental well being. Active participation also leads to a more active and productive life, not only for you the sufferer but also for your families and close ones.

10. Become Responsible

Responsibility is always difficult to achieve. It means you totally accept your feelings, thoughts and actions. It means that whether you succeed or fail, the consequences are attributable to your participation. You do not blame others, you accept feedback and see mistakes as opportunities. Responsibility also means commitment to growth at a psychological level.

Psychologically, a patient must also be well prepared to do regular exercises and take up sports/hobbies. Also important from this perspective is a realistic desire to reduce dependency on medication (in consultation with your doctor).

The so-called 'cure' is far easier to attain if you look for it within yourself. By developing these new patterns for shaping the management of your pain to your own needs, you will learn to like, accept and respect yourself. Equally you will learn to perceive yourself as being in control of your life.

These key elements will also create a more balanced commitment to relationships, work and play. As one gentleman said of our programme "It saved my marriage and family life, previously I was a total disaster to live with."

There *is* life with chronic pain. You *can* learn to manage it. That does not mean it will go away, but your tolerance can improve, so reducing the intensity of the pain. The manifestation of chronic pain can vary greatly, but to a large extent the management of that pain involves several of these key skills.

Whatever the outcome, try to be gentle with yourself.

EXERCISES

The following are illustrations and instructions for the stretches and exercises referred to in chapter 4.

Always use your pacing techniques when commencing and progressing your exercise programme.

Always warm up before exercising, and wear appropriate clothing and footwear.

To warm up correctly, you should carry out the stretches before commencing the exercises.

If an exercise causes pain, perhaps it is not appropriate for you. If in doubt, discuss with your physiotherapist or doctor.

Ideally your exercise programme should be supervised at the outset to ensure all starting positions and movements are correct. You can then continue and progress on you own.

STANDING STRETCHES

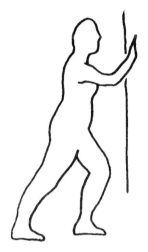

Calf Stretch

Stand about 1 foot away from a wall. Lean against it with both hands. Place one foot in front of the other, keeping the leg behind straight. Do not lift your heel off the ground. Lean forward and bend your elbows until you feel a stretch in the calf of the straight leg. Hold for 20 seconds and repeat with the opposite leg. 10 times.

Quad Stretch

Standing about 1 foot away from a wall, support yourself with your hand against the wall. Hold your opposite ankle with your other hand and bend the knee, pulling your hand towards your buttock, until you feel a stretch on the front of your thigh. Hold for 20 seconds and repeat with the opposite leg. 10 times.

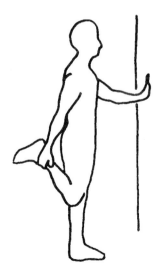

LOWER LIMB STRETCHES

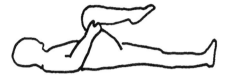

Knee to chest
Lie on your back with one leg bent. Grasp behind the knee of the bent leg and pull toward the chest. Repeat with opposite leg. Hold for 5 seconds. Repeat 15 times - progress to 25.

Hamstring stretch
Lie on your back close to a doorway. Raise one leg up onto doorway and leave the opposite leg flat. Hold for 20 seconds. Repeat with opposite leg. 10 times.

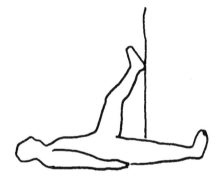

Hip Flex or Stretch
Kneel on the floor. Raise one leg with your knee bent to 90o and the foot flat on the floor. Lean forward without arching the back until you feel a stretch in the front of your thigh. Hold for 20 seconds. Repeat with the opposite leg. 10 times.

MIDDLE BACK AND NECK STRETCHES

Trunk Stretch
Sit on a chair or stool with feet well supported on floor. Raise one arm up over your head and bend sideways without lifting your buttocks off the seat. Hold for 10 seconds. Repeat with opposite side.
10 times.

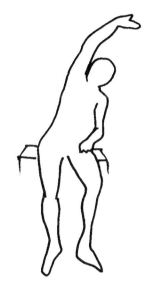

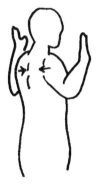

Shoulder Squeeze
Standing or sitting - raise your arms out to the side with your elbows bent at shoulder height. Push your arms backwards and squeeze your shoulderblades together. Hold for a count of 10 seconds. Repeat 10 to 15 times.

Shoulder Shrugs
Sitting or standing, squeeze shoulders up towards your ears. Hold to a count of 10 seconds, then release. Allow to relax for at least 30 seconds, and repeat 10 times. This is a good exercise to practice when you feel tension in your neck, e.g. while at the computer.

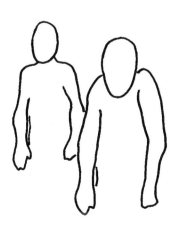

NECK EXERCISES

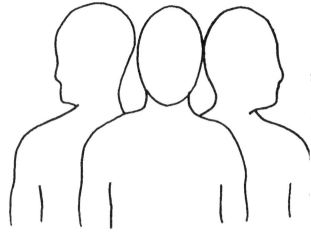

Neck Rotation
Sitting with your lower back supported, allow your head to turn slowly to the right and then to the left. Make sure your chin is parallel to the floor. Repeat 10-20 times.

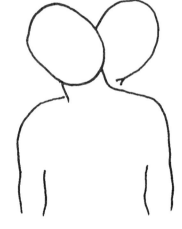

Side to Side
Sitting with your lower back supported, allow you right ear to bend towards your right shoulder. Repeat to the left. 15-20 times.

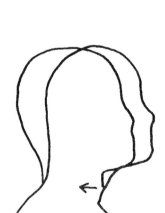

Neck Glide
Sitting as above, making sure you are looking straight ahead with your chin parallel to the floor, tuck chin in and hold for 5 seconds. Do not let your chin tilt downwards. Repeat 15 times.

LOWER BACK EXERCISES

Wall Slide
Standing with your back against a wall and with your feet a foot away from it, slide down slowly to about 45°. Hold for 10 seconds. Repeat 5 times.

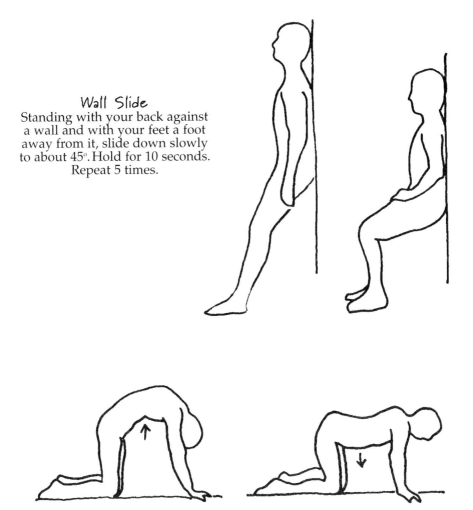

Back Press and Release
Kneeling on hands and knees, arch you back upwards, the release, allowing your stomach to fall towards the floor, and your lower back to curve downwards. Repeat 15-25 times.

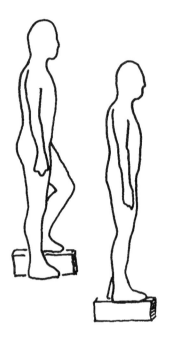

Step-ups

Use a step or equivalent. Place
the step to your left. Stand up
onto the step with your left
foot, followed by the right
foot.Repeat with opposite leg.
15-20 times.

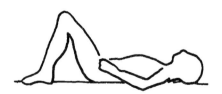

Pelvic Tilt

Lie flat on the floor with your
knees bent. Tighten your
stomach muscles and push the
curve in your lower back onto
the floor.

The following is a list of some of the places where treatment and or information is available. It is advisable first of all to contact your GP who may be able to put you in touch with a local professional or some source of help in your area.

Irish Society of Chartered Physiotherapists
Royal College of Surgeons
St Stephens Green
Dublin 2
Tel 01 478 0200 Ext. 2148

Shiatsu Society of Ireland
12 The Cave
Yellow Walls
Malahide
Co Dublin
Tel 01 845 3647

Irish Osteopathic Association
17 Windsor Terrace
Dublin 8
Tel 01 473 0828

T'ai Chi Association of Ireland
St Andrews Resource Centre
114 Pearse St
Dublin 2
Tel 01 677 1930

The Arthritis Foundation of Ireland

1 Clanwilliam Square
Grand Canal Quay
Dublin 2
Tel 01 661 8188

The Chartered Society of Physiotherapy

14 Bedford Row
London W1R 4ED
Tel 00 44 171 306 6660

The Pain Relief Foundation

Rice Lane
Liverpool L9 1AE
Tel 00 44 151 523 1486

The Pain Society
British and Irish Chapter of The IASP

9, Bedford Square
London WC1B 3RA
Tel 00 44 171 636 2750

The National Back Pain Association

16 Elmtree Rd.
Teddington
Middlesex TW11 8ST
Tel 00 44 181 977 5474

Arthritis Care

6 Grosvenor Crescent
London SW1X 7ER

The Registrar of Osteopaths

1-4 Suffolk St

London SW1

The Society of Teachers of the Alexander Technique

10 London House

266 Fulham Rd

London SW10

Society of Homeopaths

2 Artisaw Rd

Northampton

American Pain Society

340 Kingsland St

Nutley

NJ 07110, USA

International Association for The Study of Pain

909 NE 43rd St.

Suite 306

Seattle, WA 98105-6020, USA

Irish Psychological Society

13 Adelaide Rd

Dublin 2

Tel 01 783 916

Back Pain Association

Grundy House

31-33 Park Rd

Teddington

Middlesex TW17 OAB

RECOMMENDED READING

Back Care, The Health Promotion Unit, Ireland.

The Readers Digest Guide to Alternative Medicine, Consumers Association.

Migraine and Headaches - Understanding, Controlling and Avoiding the Pain.
Wilkinson, M, Martin Dunitz, London 1982.

Life After Stress.
Shaffer, M, Contemporary Books Inc., Chicago 1983.

Stresswise - A Practical Guide for Dealing with Stress.
Looker, T, Gregson, O, Hodder and Stoughton, U.K. 1989.

The Back - Relief from Pain.
Stoddard, A, Martin Dunitz, London 1982.

Conquering Pain.
Lipton, S, Martin Dunitz, London 1984.

Living With Your Pain.
Broome, A, Jellicoe, H, Methuen, London, 1987.

Conquering Pain
Forest, JB, Empowering Press, Hamilton, Canada 1994.

The Joy of Stress
Hanson, P, Cox and Wyman Ltd., Reading, 1986

Natural Therapies, The Complete A-Z Guide of Complementary Health.
McCarthy, M, Thorsons, Harper Collins, 1994.

You Can Heal Your Life.
Hay, Louise L, Eden Grove, London 1984.

The Doctors Guide to Instant Stress Relief.
Nathan, R.G., Ballantine Books, N.Y., 1987.

Thoughts and Feelings - The Art of Cognitive Stress Intervention.
McKay, M, Davis M, Fanning P, New Harbinger Publications, USA 1981.

The Relaxation and Stress Reduction Workbook.
Davis, M, Robbins Eshelman, E, McKay M, New Harbinger Publications, USA, 1991

Psychological Approaches to Pain Management - A Practitioners Handbook.
Gatchel, R.J., Turk, D.C., Guildford Press N.Y. 1996.

When Ill-Health Becomes Your Enemy.
Moore-Groarke, G, Thompson, S, Mercier Press, Cork 1996.

The Pain Relief Handbook
Wells, C, Nown, G, Vermilion, London, 1996.

The Challenge of Pain
R. Melzack & P. D Wall, Penguin.

The Puzzle of Pain
Melzack, Penguin.

INDEX

The Authors

Jack Barrett MB, Bch, BAO, FFARCSI

Qualified UCC 1975. Specialised in Anaesthesia. Has worked as part of his anaesthetic practice in pain clinics since 1978. Returned to Ireland in 1986. Set up *Pain Management Centre* in Douglas, Cork in 1997. The speciality of Anaesthesia has been a driving force behind the development of pain management for the past 25 years.

Marna Carey MCSP

Qualified as a physiotherapist in 1982 from Queen Margaret College, Edinburgh. Worked in Dumfries and Glasgow before going to Australia. Travelled and worked in various locations. Set up private practice in Sydney - providers for a small general hospital where experience was gained in rehabilitation and out-patients. Developed an interest in chronic pain and gained a diploma in Shiatsu. Returned to Cork in 1995. Worked in private practice and out-patients, and joined the *Pain Management Centre* in 1997. Member of the Chartered Society of Physiotherapists.

Gillian Moore-Groarke BA(Hons), PhD, NUI, Reg. Psychol. APsSI

Qualified with a PhD in Health Psychology in 1990. Worked as a director/consultant psychologist as part of St Francis Medical Centre until setting up private practice in 1996. She is a registered psychologist and has been a part-time lecturer in UCC from 1990-1998. Author of a number of books including the best selling *"When Food Becomes Your Enemy"* She contributes regularly to radio and television on issues relating to health psychology. Columnist Cork Examiner 1998. Has worked with Jack Barrett since opening private practice in 1996. Joined *Pain Management Centre* in 1997. Her interest in health psychology has been the main contributing force in her interest in pain management. She is also an advisor to *Weight Watchers* international professional/advisory board.

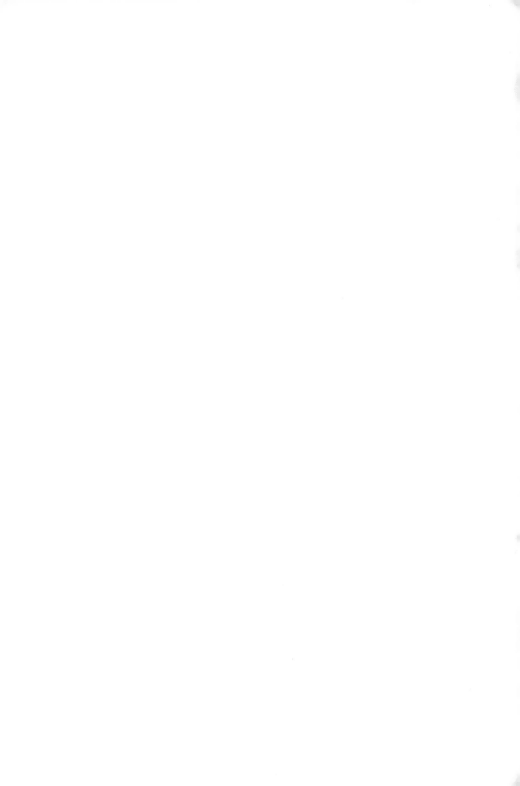